BECOMING A DAD

The First-Time Dad's Guide To Pregnancy Preparation (101 Tips For Expectant Dads)

LISA MARSHALL
JOHNNY ANTONELLI

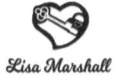

CONTENTS

Introduction	xi
1. You're Having a Baby!	1
2. Getting Ready to Be Parents	9
3. Talking About The Future	13
4. Early Preparations	19
5. Finances	25
6. Preparing Your Home	33
7. First Trimester - Conception Through 12 Weeks	41
8. Second Trimester - 13 to 27 Weeks	49
9. Third Trimester - 28 to 40 Weeks	57
10. Complications in Pregnancy	67
11. Going Into Labor	77
12. Who's Going to Be There When The Baby Comes?	81
13. Childbirth Methods And Gear	85
14. Complications in Labor And Childbirth	91
15. The Birth Itself	97
16. Cesarean Section	107
17. Complications After Delivery	113
18. Now You Have a Baby!	115
19. Baby Care at Home	123
20. Parental Care at Home	131
Conclusion	137
Thank You	141
Also by Lisa Marshall	143

Copyright © 2019 by Lisa Marshall - All rights reserved.

No part of this publication may be reproduced, stored in a retrieval system, or transmitted in any form or by any means, electronic, mechanical, photocopying, recording, scanning, or otherwise, except as permitted under Sections 107 or 108 of the 1976 United States Copyright Act, without the prior written permission of the Publisher. Requests to the Publisher for permission should be addressed to the Permission Department, Newcommunicationline Press, Pod. S. Giovanna d'Arco 1, 58044 Cinigiano (GR), Italy.

Limit of Liability/Disclaimer of Warranty: The Publisher and the author make no representations of warranties with respect to the accuracy or completeness of the contents of this work and specifically disclaim all warranties, including without limitation warranties of fitness for a particular purpose. No warranty may be created or extended by sales or promotional materials. The advice and strategies contained herein may not be suitable for every situation. This work is sold with the understanding that the Publisher is not engaged in rendering medical, legal, or other professional advice or services. If professional assistance is required, the services of a competent professional person should be sought. Neither the Publisher nor the author shall be liable for damages arising therefrom. The fact that an individual, organization, or website is referred to in this work as a citation and/or potential source of further information does not mean that the author or the Publisher endorses the information the individual, organization, or website may provide or recommendations they/it may make. Further, readers should be aware that Internet websites listed in this work was written and when it is read.

For general information on our other products and services or to obtain technical support, please contact info@newcommunbicationline.com

Newcommunicationline Press publishes its books in a variety of electronic and print formats. Some content that appears in print may not be available in electronic books, and vice versa.

TRADEMARKS: Newcommunicationline Press and the Newcommunicationline Press Logo are trademarks of Giovanni Antonelli and may not be used without permission. All other trademarks are the property of their respective owners.

Lisa Marshall

lisamarshall@newcommuniactionline.com

www.facebook.com/LisaMarshallAuthor

ISBN 978-1650917672

ISBN 978-1690437109

ISBN 978-1690437086

ASIN B0834B1GMQ

10 9 8 7 6 5 4 3 2 1

YOUR FREE GIFT

As a way of saying thanks for your purchase, I wanted to offer you a free bonus. This tool is a useful handbook with quick tips to help you know what to expect during pregnancy and how you can help...

To get instant access just tap here or go to:

http://bit.ly/survivalguidefordadstobe

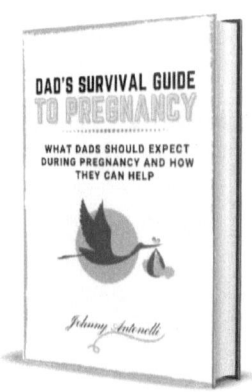

Inside this survival guide:

- Find out what to expect month by month.
- Get fast tips on how to support your partner.
- Everything you need to know about pregnancy.

DO YOU ENJOY AUDIOBOOKS ?

If you prefer to learn by listening, be sure to check out my audiobooks! You can listen for FREE if you're a first time Audible user as part of their free 30-day trial.
Click the link below and enjoy your next audiobook...

>> https://bit.ly/enjoyaudiobooks <<

Now "*Becoming A Dad*" audiobook version is also available!

DAD...
"A SON'S FIRST HERO, A DAUGHTER'S FIRST LOVE"

— JOHNNY ANTONELLI

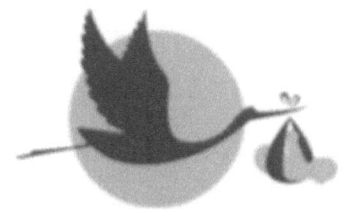

INTRODUCTION

By Johnny Antonelli

"Wait, What! I'm gonna be a dad?!"

Most probably, it is the reaction you tend to give when you hear about wife's pregnancy news. A single sentence has freaked you out and a lot of thoughts are going through your mind.

You cannot figure out whether you are feeling happy, emotional, or fearful. It's normal, as we all go through the same emotions. You may be worried about how you will support your partner during pregnancy and childbirth, especially how your new baby is going to change your lifestyle. It feels like a huge responsibility and you start to surf the internet looking for advice for expecting dads.

The end result would be a huge amount of contrasting information that will make you more confused. I know this because it has happened to me too. But don't worry! We got you.

This book provides advice and tips for expectant dads, focusing on what to do during pregnancy, childbirth, and just after the baby is born. I have created this book with my friend and parenting expert, Lisa Marshall, so you can have a reliable source of information.

Hence, this step-by-step guide to pregnancy preparation for dads-to-be will give you authentic tips from the expert. Given my personal experience, at the beginning, I did not have any idea about how to take care of a baby. I was scared! I didn't even know how to feed a baby or how to make them fall asleep. Nonetheless, these responsibilities will come later. Another immediate concern was the pregnancy phase. I had no clue how the mother would feel about the changes and how I could support her.

Considering all these points, we have included all the pregnancy phases, relevant tips, and complications.

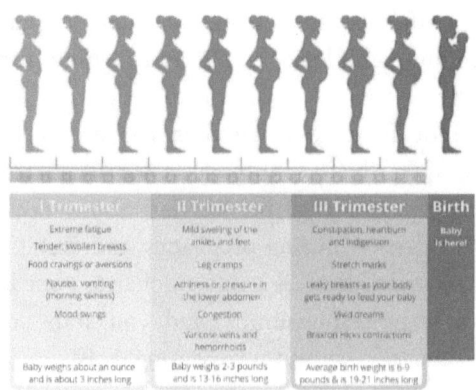

Each trimester of pregnancy brings new experiences, changes and challenges - for mama and baby.

It is common that you will be worried about financial management from the moment you hear this news. Generally, income is the primary source of conflict between partners.

Hence, you have to plan the finances with your partner in the initial days and consider the ways you can start saving money for the baby, which is discussed in the book.

Besides, the book also covers the ways and tips to prepare the home for the baby. During and even after pregnancy, a woman goes through a lot of physical and hormonal changes in her body. She needs your support, considering the physical and emotional stress she is going through. Also, you will find guidance about how to be there for your partner and help her.

Pregnancy is a matter of two and it is essential that the father is involved from the first moment and goes with the future mother to medical visits, childbirth preparation courses, and to help her as much as possible so that he begins to live parenthood from the beginning.

FETAL GROWTH FROM 4 TO 40 WEEKS

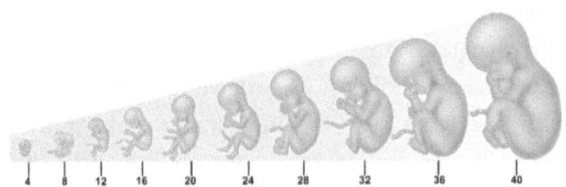

I know that when you broke the news that your wife was pregnant, you were basically telling everyone "*We are pregnant.*"

Weeks go by, you begin to realize that, logically, she is the pregnant woman. Also, there are moments when you begin to feel that things are not going as planned with you. We, dads, have it a bit bad because we do not feel the baby, we do not notice it, and we only know it when the child is born.

Hence, we offer you some tips briefly so that you can get the feel of the book and be able to be involved during pregnancy and feel a bit yours too.

1. Communicate more than ever – You are about to experience one of the biggest changes a couple can experience. So, it is very important that you talk about it. Ask her how she feels and talk about the baby, the changes in your lives, and the additional one more member in your lives. Talking about these things will help in visualizing how you see yourselves in the parenthood role and the expectations related to it.

2. Visit the gynecologist and midwife together – Even though your partner is the pregnant woman, you can also become aware of the progression of fetal growth. Take advantage of the moments when you will get the first-hand news about the evolution of the baby. During visits, you will be able to see your baby in the ultrasounds and hear the heartbeat and know what the health professional thinks about the progress. You will learn about the precautions or advice that the gynecologist might give for better outcomes.

3. Change with her – Women start to take more care of themselves during pregnancy by eating a healthy, balanced diet and doing regular exercise. You can encourage her by getting involved with her so that your partner feels that you are "there" for her. There is a specific section related to diet and exercise that can enlighten you about the types of exercise that will benefit the mother.

4. Become parents together – Becoming parents of a child is one of the greatest responsibilities adults can have. Thus, it is necessary to be prepared for this as much as possible, so that you are ensured you are on the right path. For this purpose, you can read this comprehensive book and discuss it with your partner, rather than reading unreliable and confusing information from different sources. In this way, both of you will learn from the book and also understand each other's perspectives.

5. Connect with the baby – It is difficult to have contact with the baby because it inside your partner's belly. However, you can try to connect with the baby by talking to him/her, singing, and touching the belly to feel the baby. The movements become more evident as the weeks go by and you will be able to feel parts of the baby's body. Believe me, it is not little! Putting your hand and noticing how it moves in your palm is not little and can go as far to build a connection.

6. Doing preparations and shopping together – Discuss with your partner the things that will be bought for the baby and make room for them. Do the shopping together to buy things that will suit your home and taste. Start learning how things work, so you can take care of the baby alone and do not put all the burden on the mother. This book can be a helpful tool to learn about how to take care of the baby.

Recent studies on parenthood and baby health have shown that the role of a father is as important as the mother; hence, you have to be prepared for the experience of fatherhood. The purpose is to give you insights to be prepared for pregnancy and the birth of a child clearly and sensibly.

What makes this book different from the others? **Why is it so special?**

It is because we have included the process from the perspective of both, moms and dads.

Two viewpoints will offer an overall experience behind this wonderful but complex walk with your partner.

Before starting this adventure, I would like to give a brief review of the information that you will gather from this book.

You are going to discover:

- What each trimester will bring in terms of physical, medical, and hormonal experience, with emphasis on the prenatal care required for each trimester.
- What are the symptoms of some of the common complications in pregnancy. Remember that you probably won't be dealing with any of the complications, but having knowledge might help in detecting the problem early if there is any.
- The ways you can support your partner during the emotional ups and downs because hormones cause sudden mood swings. You have to understand and deal with them even if it is a bit complicated. Besides, it is normal that your partner will feel more exhausted, so you can take care of the household chores and other work that she does to help her ease off stress.
- A detailed insight into what labor stages your partner will go through and who will be present in the labor room when the baby comes. Besides, it includes childbirth methods and the complications associated with labor and childbirth and after delivery.
- The detailed information regarding the initial nursing guide and the medications the baby will receive before going home.
- How the parents can manage the finances and insurances, prepare the home for the child, and change the dietary and physical activity plans.

- The reality when you are home looking after the baby and dealing with the emotional and physical stress of your partner. The guide will prepare you to be able to handle the situation with patience and understanding.

Remember, the baby will come in your life after nine months and till then, you have to cherish the process of pregnancy and what your partner is going through for the baby. The intent to learn about pregnancy and fatherhood implies that you are on the right path to becoming a dad. By the way, it is vital that you learn continuously throughout parenthood.

In all cases, this guide will be a fruitful ride for expectant dads, as they will discover new things every step of the way.

If you did not yet, I highly suggest you download the mini-guide at the beginning of the book in "your free gift" section. It is a survival handbook for dads-to-be, very useful whenever you need quick solutions.

So, it's time to dive into the book!

You are going to be a father and you will have an amazing journey ahead.

Chapter One
YOU'RE HAVING A BABY!

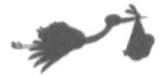

There are two kinds of pregnancies: The planned, and the unplanned.

If you and your partner have been trying to get pregnant—congrats! You're embarking on life's greatest adventure together.

And if you and your partner have been trying *not* to get pregnant—still congrats! You might not have thought you were ready yet, but it's still going to be an adventure.

Planned or unplanned, finding out you have a baby on the way is just the first step on a journey that will take you places you never imagined. But no need to panic! Generations of men before you have become dads and lived to tell the tale. You can do this, too. This book will cover everything you need to know about pregnancy, childbirth and what comes afterward.

The key is to know something about what's going to happen next, so you can get ready. Sure, your partner is doing the heavy lifting physically, but you're in this together and your participation is mission-critical. So strap in, because it's gonna be a bumpy ride. But the payoff is unbelievable.

HOW DO YOU KNOW SHE'S PREGNANT?

Most likely your partner purchased a home pregnancy test. When she opened the box she found a stick that looked something like a digital thermometer. She was instructed to pee on the stick, wait a few minutes, and check the little window. The window might show lines, or negative or positive signs, or even the words "pregnant" or "not pregnant."

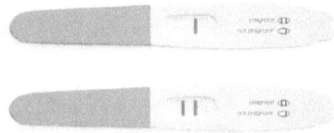

This kind of pregnancy test works by checking the urine for a hormone called human chorionic gonadotropin (hCG). When a fertilized egg settles into the uterus, the cells that will become the placenta start making this hormone. The amount of hCG being made doubles every 72 hours up until about 12 weeks into pregnancy. By the time your partner realized her period was late, there was enough hCG in her urine to show up on a home pregnancy test.

Are home pregnancy tests always accurate?

Pregnancy tests are pretty darn accurate, but nothing in life is 100%.

In the early days of home pregnancy tests, a woman had to wait until her period was at least a couple of weeks late. Then, she had to limit how much she drank the night before and test her urine first thing in the morning. That was all to make sure the level of hCG in her urine was high enough for the test.

Now, she can test on the day her period should start (possibly even before) and she can do the test any time of day. This is because the technology for detecting hCG has become extremely sensitive.

However, tests results aren't accurate every single time. It isn't common, but there can be both false negatives (she's pregnant, but the test says she isn't) and false positives (she's not pregnant, but the test says she is).

What causes a false negative?

A negative result can be disappointing—or a huge relief. It can also be inaccurate, if the woman is pregnant but there's not enough hCG in her urine for the test to pick up on. While today's tests are way more sensitive than they were in the past, they still have limits.

It's important to read the instructions that come with the test. She can get a false negative if she takes the test too soon, if her urine is too diluted or if she just doesn't wait long enough to check the stick for the result.

What causes a false positive?

A positive result can bring joy or sorrow. But again, while they are even less common than false negatives, false positives can occur.

Many pregnancies end early, even before the woman suspects she is pregnant. The fertilized egg may have attached to the uterus but for some reason just didn't take. An early test may pick up on hCG from a pregnancy that has already ended.

Sometimes a fertilized egg attaches someplace outside the uterus, in what's known as an ectopic pregnancy. Ectopic pregnancies can go away on their own, but often they have to be removed surgically because they can be life-threatening for the woman.

Some medications can cause false positive results. This obviously includes hormone treatments, but it also includes a few that might surprise you, like methadone and some antidepressants.

Some medical conditions can lead to false positives, especially if they cause white or red blood cells to show up in the urine.

How do you confirm a home pregnancy test result?

If the result is positive, or if it's negative but your partner still thinks she might be pregnant, she can always wait a week or two and take another test. Many tests come in packages of two for just this reason.

However, if she's having worrisome symptoms like pain or unusual bleeding, or if it's important to know about a pregnancy as soon as possible, she can see a healthcare provider for confirmation. She can see her regular primary care provider or go to a Planned Parenthood clinic. She should be cautious about going to a "crisis pregnancy center" as these places often provide inaccurate or incomplete information.

Most healthcare providers test urine using the very same technology as home pregnancy tests. They don't usually do blood tests for pregnancy, but they may do them for other reasons.

Depending on how far along the pregnancy is thought to be, a physical exam may be done. They may have your partner lay down on an examining table, then press on her belly to see if her uterus is enlarged. They may do an internal exam to look at her cervix, the lower part of her uterus. In pregnancy the cervix will soften and change color.

If the pregnancy is far enough along, they may check for a heartbeat. After about 10 weeks it may be possible to pick up the baby's heartbeat with a handheld device called a Doppler, which is kind of like an audio-only ultrasound. Some midwives like to go old school with a Pinard horn, an ancient kind of stethoscope that looks something like a really skinny Pilsner glass.

And of course, for the ultimate audio-visual experience, they may do an ultrasound. Early on, six to eight weeks or so, ultrasounds are usually done trans-vaginally, with a slender device inserted into the vagina. Not every woman is going to be okay with that, and it isn't usually done unless there's an important reason for it.

Otherwise, she is likely to be offered a trans-abdominal ultrasound at around 12 weeks. This is the less-intrusive kind they show on TV, where the device is passed over her belly. At this early stage you'll definitely hear a heartbeat but the visuals may be hard to figure out. Sometimes you see something that really looks like a baby, but sometimes it's a lot of static and you have to take the technician's word for it!

The ultimate in ultrasound tech is the 3D format. It produces a picture that's so eerily lifelike it almost feels voyeuristic, like you should give the little guy some privacy. (But instead, it'll probably go straight to Instagram.)

WHAT ARE THE SYMPTOMS OF EARLY PREGNANCY?

Long before she starts looking pregnant, your partner will start feeling the effects of the flow of pregnancy hormones. Typical symptoms include:

- Nausea, sometimes with vomiting
- Feeling bloated and gassy
- Very tender breasts
- Fatigue
- Sensitivity to smells and tastes that didn't bother her before
- Headaches
- Feeling emotional

This may not sound like much fun, and for many women it really isn't much fun. Fortunately, she should start feeling better within a few weeks.

Typically, pregnancy lasts about nine calendar months, and it's divided into three parts, called trimesters. An old saying, "Three months dreary, three months cheery and three months weary," describes it pretty well.

During those first three months—the first trimester—your partner may feel tired, cranky and weepy. In the second trimester the earlier discomforts usually start to resolve, and she may start to really enjoy being pregnant. Her energy comes back, she enjoys food again and she has a proud little baby bump. In the last trimester she may start having new discomforts owing to the size of the baby and its weight as it presses on her bladder and diaphragm, and she might start counting the days until the baby comes and she has her body back.

More about all of this soon.

WHAT IF THE PREGNANCY FAILS?

When a pregnancy ends unexpectedly before 20 weeks, this is known as a miscarriage. About 10 percent to 20 percent of known pregnancies end in miscarriage, usually in the first trimester. After 12 weeks the risk of miscarriage decreases dramatically. This is why many couples will wait until 12 weeks to start telling friends and family that they're expecting.

It's estimated that about 50 percent to 75 percent of pregnancies actually end before the woman even knows she's pregnant. When this happens, her period is usually on time or perhaps a little late. She may or may not have more cramping than usual.

Having a miscarriage after the pregnancy has been confirmed can cause emotions from sadness to devastation, depending on how much it was wanted. Even if the pregnancy was unintended and neither of you were really happy about it, you might find an early miscarriage leaves you with a surprising mixture of relief and sadness.

If you've told others that you were expecting, you may dread having to now tell them there's not going to be a baby after all. This can be hard to do, but may also bring some comfort. It is very likely that many women you know have had miscarriages they never talked about; they'll talk about them now, and you'll realize how common this experience really is.

Chapter Two

GETTING READY TO BE PARENTS

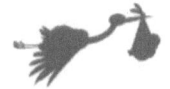

When you were a kid, *parents* were old people of an earlier generation. They were adults and they did adult stuff, like going to work, and mowing the lawn, and never running out of toilet paper. It might be impossible to imagine your parents as a young couple, living wild and free. But what you are now, they once were—and what they are now, you will be. Impossible, right? Yeah, that's what your dad thought, too, when he was in your shoes.

You're going to be a dad. And your partner is going to be a mom—if you feel intimidated, imagine how she feels! Fortunately, you're a team. You're going to figure this out together.

First, though, to be the best parents you can be you need to make sure you take care of yourselves and each other. Before getting into the details of parenthood, let's talk about how to protect and strengthen your relationship.

TAKING A BABYMOON

WHAT'S A BABYMOON?

If you're married, you may or may not have had a honeymoon—time away, just the two of you, to revel in your new status. Back in the day, getting married meant spending nights alone together for the first time. A honeymoon was important for figuring out how to be a couple.

Nowadays most couples have spent nights together before the wedding; in fact, they have likely lived together. A honeymoon is still nice, though, because being married is still a change from not being married.

A babymoon is based on the same kind of idea. However long you've been together, becoming parents means a dramatic change in your relationship. What you're gaining will far outweigh what you're losing, but one part of your life is ending forever: the part where it's just the two of you. A babymoon is a celebration of both the life you're leaving behind and the life you're about to begin.

How long should a babymoon be?

This is entirely up to you. If you want to take your dream trip together, go for it. If you are limited by time and money, keep it simple. Some couples will check off an exotic bucket-list destination, and some will spend a quiet weekend not too far from home. The point is to be together, knowing that big changes are coming.

When should you take your babymoon?

Again, this is up to you. Besides practicalities of time and money, consider the physical demands of pregnancy. If you want to go on a long journey, engage in strenuous activities or go where medical care is not readily available, you'll probably want to aim for the second trimester, between 12 and 20 weeks. That way you'll be past the discomforts of early pregnancy and highest risk of miscarriage, and not yet into the discomforts of late pregnancy or chance of early labor.

If you're going for a quiet weekend close to home and you want to have your babymoon nearer to the baby's arrival, you can wait until the last trimester. At that point you'll be very aware of the huge leap you're about to take together, and this time together can feel especially meaningful.

SEX

Do you both love spontaneous romantic gestures? Still savor wild, passionate nights and long, lazy mornings in bed? Have just a few spots left in the house where you haven't enjoyed an unplanned quickie?

No one's saying you can't have any of that after the baby comes. It's just that you probably won't—not for a while, at least. It's okay, that's normal.

But what about sex while your partner is pregnant?

IS IT OKAY TO HAVE SEX DURING PREGNANCY?

In rare cases, there may be complications with a pregnancy that puts sex off limits, at least for some period of time. But for the most part, sex is perfectly safe for the baby, even late into the third trimester. If babies in the uterus could not survive the normal activities of mom's daily life, humans would have died out long ago.

Generally speaking, the only thing limiting your sexual activity is how sexy you and your partner feel. This is likely to change throughout the pregnancy, and you may not always be in sync. Sometimes you'll be turned on by her growing breasts, but they'll be so sore she can't stand for you to touch them. Sometimes her surging hormones will make her super horny, but feeling the baby move as she pulls you closer makes you go limp.

As with every aspect of your relationship, honesty (and a sense of humor) is critical. Talk to each other, take it day by day, and don't compare yourself to what others say they're doing.

Chapter Three

TALKING ABOUT THE FUTURE

Maybe you were one of those couples who found out on the first date that your parenting philosophies were in perfect sync. Maybe you both came from loving, healthy families. Maybe your own parents were such excellent role models you know exactly how it all works.

Or maybe when you first starting dating neither of you had ever imagined having kids of your own. Maybe your own parents weren't such great role models, and most of what you learned from them was what *not* to do. Maybe now that a baby is on the way, you're beginning to suspect you're not on the same page at all.

Life doesn't always proceed according to plan, and not all the decisions you make are going to pan out. There will be unforeseen twists and turns, and from time to time you'll need to rethink how you thought things would go.

Your feelings, and your partner's feelings, about many aspects of parenting will change with time and experience. The key to parenting, as with so many other things in life, is to have a plan— while remaining flexible.

SOME THINGS TO CONSIDER—FOR NOW

WILL ONE (OR BOTH) OF YOU STAY HOME?

Do you have the luxury of allowing one of you to stay home full-time with the baby? If so, who will it be? Will you take turns? Keep in mind that caring for an infant is a full-time job in itself. Trying to work from home while being solely responsible for the baby's care can be far more difficult than you might imagine. At least in the beginning, plan to keep baby care and work separate.

If either or both of you have jobs that offer paid parental leave, take it! In some fields it might mean your career trajectory takes a hit, but this is changing. And you know it's true that no one ever lays on their death bed wishing they'd spent more time at the office. Getting paid to stay home with your new family is a given in some cultures, but in others it's a rare gift to be treasured.

WILL YOU USE DAYCARE?

At some point you may both need to return to work. Can you arrange your schedules so one of you is always with the baby? This may seem like the ideal arrangement, but if either or both of you work outside the home, it may mean you never see each other during waking hours. That can take a serious toll on your relationship.

The alternative is to have someone else look after the baby while you both work. Unless you have family willing and able to do this, it means hiring someone. Will you get a nanny or au pair who comes to your home? Will you drop the baby off at daycare? Will it be licensed daycare in someone else's home, or at a commercial daycare center? Do either of your workplaces offer childcare?

Of course, while considering your options you'll need to

take into account how much childcare will cost. Full-time daycare can be shockingly expensive! You may find it's actually more affordable for one of you to stay home, at least for a while. In any case, it's important to discuss these topics openly and be on the same page.

HOW WILL HOUSEHOLD DUTIES BE SHARED?

Ever see one of those old TV shows where the husband complains he works hard all day while the wife gets to stay home and chill, while the wife complains the husband gets to kick back in the office all day while she works her fingers to the bone? Then they swap places, and neither can handle what the other does?

Reality is, of course, somewhere in the middle. Maybe you can't wait to go to work each day, and you come home feeling refreshed and energetic. Or maybe you come home feeling exhausted and brain-dead, craving a cold beer and some mindless TV. Either way, you might feel you've done enough for the day and deserve some time off.

But if you've ever been the partner at home with the baby all day, you know full-on parenting is at least as exhausting as working outside the home. When your partner walks in the door at the end of the day you may be ready to hand over that baby and head for the hills.

And yet, stuff still needs to be done. Cooking, dishes, laundry, oil changes . . . unless you are lucky enough to have hired help, it's up to the two of you. The time to figure out who's going to do what is now, not when you find yourself in crisis.

SOME THINGS TO CONSIDER—FOR LATER

As your child grows, there will be more decisions to be made. You don't have to settle these right now, but start the conversation now so to avoid surprises later.

WHAT'S YOUR PHILOSOPHY ON DISCIPLINE?

This is likely to be based on your own upbringing, whether you want to follow your parents' example or defy it, and the same will be true for your partner.

Some children are so naturally well-behaved they need little in the way of guidance, but what if yours is a hellion? How will you handle defiance and misbehavior? Do you believe in spanking? Time-outs? Withholding allowance or favorite activities? Can you control your own temper when dealing with a misbehaving child?

If you want to know more about discipline, you can find a lot of useful and effective tips on my book " Toddler Discipline Tips" - The Complete Parenting Guide With Proven Strategies To Understand And Managing Toddler's Behavior, Dealing With Tantrums, And Reach An Effective Communications With Kids.

WHAT KIND OF SCHOOLING DO YOU WANT YOUR CHILD TO HAVE?

There are so many choices! Public school, private school, parochial school, homeschooling, unschooling, online schooling . . . Where your child ends up will to some degree depend on his or her personality, interests and abilities, but you and your partner are bound to have some strong feelings about how you want your child educated.

. . .

How will you approach gender expectations?

When you were a kid, gender differences were probably pretty well defined. Even with a liberal upbringing, boys were boys and girls were girls. Clothing stores, toy aisles and recess activities were clearly segregated. There were two genders, and everyone identified as one or the other.

Whether you find it liberating or distressing, gender roles and expectations—even the very definition of gender—are changing. At the same time, Instagram is overflowing with expectant parents outdoing each other in the scale of their gender-reveal parties. People are still going to ask you if you're having boy or a girl.

Do you want to find out the sex of your baby before its born? Are you going to buy clothing and decorations that are pink and frilly, or blue and bold? Or are you going to decorate and buy newborn outfits in neutral yellows and greens and be surprised when the baby comes?

And once you know, what then? Are you going to encourage your daughter to take ballet, or your son to play football? Are you going to leave all options on the table and let them decide? What if they don't know if they want to be a boy or a girl? Or they identify as something that doesn't match their genitals? What if your child is intersex, and not clearly either male or female?

Of course, you won't have answers for all these questions immediately. Some will be easier to answer when you know your child better, and some will, in time, answer themselves. What's important now is to talk about how you'll approach these sensitive issues, and how you'll support your child regardless of gender.

What about healthcare matters?

This used to be a no-brainer. Boys were circumcised, or

not, depending largely on family tradition. Everyone followed the recommended vaccination schedule, and everyone who had access to regular dental care got routine X-rays, fillings and fluoride treatments.

Nowadays, though, parents are less likely to accept conventional wisdom without asking questions. You and your partner will want to make well-informed decisions about your child's health, but it will be challenging to know if you're getting reliable information. Now is the time to see where you both stand on healthcare matters, and to agree on trusted sources you'll turn to when you need to know more.

Chapter Four
EARLY PREPARATIONS

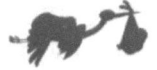

DIET

*I*s a pregnant woman "eating for two?" Kind of . . . but not really.

In the first trimester, a woman doesn't usually need to take in any extra calories. The baby-to-be is just an embryo at this stage and doesn't need a lot in the way of building materials. If she has morning sickness or is having trouble handling the way things taste, she should eat what she can.

In the second and third trimesters she needs to take in about 400 to 500 extra calories per day. Those extra calories can come from larger portions of her regular meals, or from healthy between-meal snacks. Many women find several small meals each day sit better with them than a few large ones, especially as the baby grows and begins pressing on her internal organs.

A woman can follow any kind of diet that provides the nutrients she and the baby need. "Diet" means vegan, vegetarian, flexitarian, omnivore, etc. It definitely does not mean weight-loss! If your partner is overweight when she gets pregnant she may be advised to limit how much she gains, but this is not the time to try to lose weight.

Prenatal vitamins

Most women will take a prenatal vitamin while pregnant. If the pregnancy was planned, she may have started taking vitamins while trying to conceive. She may well continue taking them after the baby is born, too, especially if she breastfeeds.

Prenatal vitamins contain all the nutrients found in regular multivitamins plus some that are especially important in pregnancy. Most prenatal vitamins have iron, for example, to help keep mom from becoming anemic. Anemia, or not enough red blood cells, is common in pregnancy because so many more are needed to make sure the baby is getting its share. Another critical nutrient is folic acid, which helps prevent birth defects in the baby's brain and spine.

Alcohol

The advice women have been given over the years about drinking during pregnancy has varied. We know that when a pregnant woman drinks, some alcohol reaches the baby. We know alcohol can contribute to miscarriage, stillbirth and health problems in the baby. What we don't know is how much alcohol it takes to cause these problems.

The current medical consensus is that there is no amount of alcohol that is known to be safe during pregnancy, nor any stage of pregnancy when it's known to be safe to drink. Therefore, women who are pregnant, or trying to become pregnant, are advised to avoid alcohol altogether.

Obviously, this isn't a problem if your partner doesn't

drink anyway. If she does drink regularly—especially if she has trouble limiting how much she drinks—this will present a special challenge.

Heavy drinking during pregnancy can cause severe, lifelong disability in your child. These disabilities are now known as fetal alcohol spectrum disorders (FASDs) and include problems with vision and hearing, low IQ, learning disabilities, ADHD and problems with the heart and kidneys, among many others.

If your partner drinks, make sure she understands the risks this presents. Trying to police and control her behavior is unlikely to be successful, and may just strain your relationship. Suggest she talk to her doctor, midwife or other healthcare provider about getting help. Perhaps she'll be willing to try AA.

You can help make this easier for her by also giving up alcohol until the baby comes. Look for non-alcoholic alternatives to the drinks you both enjoy, and be sure to bring them along to social gatherings where alcohol will be served.

MERCURY

Not all forms of mercury are equally toxic. The kind that becomes an issue in pregnancy is called methylmercury, which can cross the placenta and cause serious injury to the developing baby. Methylmercury finds its way into the ocean both through natural processes and through human activity. This most dangerous form of mercury can accumulate in large predatory fish like sharks, swordfish and king mackerel, and pregnant women should avoid eating these. Other kinds of seafood like shrimp, salmon and albacore tuna are less likely to contain dangerous amounts of methylmercury and may be eaten in moderation. Of course, there's no problem here if your partner doesn't care for seafood anyway.

EXERCISE

Regular exercise is important during pregnancy, both to maintain mental and physical fitness and to prepare for childbirth. If your partner was very active before she got pregnant she will probably want to stay active now. If she didn't get much exercise before it may be a challenge, but all three of you will be better off if she gets up and moving. If she ends up on bedrest or has physical disabilities that limit her mobility, she'll need some expert advise on how to stay fit.

Early pregnancy often brings nausea (and sometimes vomiting) and fatigue. Your partner may also find her stamina lagging and have trouble with activities that demand cardiovascular fitness, like cycling, running and cross-country skiing. This can be frustrating for both of you, but you can usually look forward to the return of her normal energy level once she's out of the first trimester. In late pregnancy, of course, she may have to cut back on some activities as the size of her belly and the change in her center of gravity require some adjustments.

Swimming can be a great form of exercise that easily accommodates her changing body. Depending on where you live there may be yoga, pilates and other exercise classes specifically designed for pregnant women. The ultimate form of exercise for the pregnant woman though (assuming her mobility is not otherwise limited), is walking.

Walking can be relaxing or invigorating—or both! It's good for heart, lungs, bones and muscles and can clear her head and lift her mood. It's especially beneficial to the muscles she'll be using during childbirth; in fact, she will likely be encouraged to keep walking while she's in labor. You can do your part by going with her or, if she's really craving some time to herself, helping clear her schedule so she can get out on her own.

ARE THERE ANY KINDS OF EXERCISE SHE CAN'T DO?
You're likely to hear a lot of advice and opinions on what kinds of physical activity a pregnant woman should or shouldn't engage in. This is very individual, and common-sense, fitness level and previous experience will be determining factors. Pregnancy is probably not the time to take up water skiing or horseback riding, for example, but if these are activities she loves and does well, she probably won't want to give them up. Some woman run marathons—and even triathlons—while pregnant!

Of course, unexpected complications can end up limiting how much she can do, and even the most fit woman is likely to reach a point where the physical demands of pregnancy force her to slow down a bit.

Chapter Five
FINANCES

Nothing brings financial matters into focus like impending parenthood. Whether by nature you're a spender or a saver, a planner or a freewheeler, decisions must be made. As with everything involved in getting ready for your first child, the key is to have a plan while remaining flexible—because nothing ever goes according to plan.

Money is the number one source of conflict between partners of all kinds, and fighting over finances can be a relationship killer. Talk about this stuff now, make a plan, and get on the same page. It's important for all three of you.

PARENTAL LEAVE

(This is for informational purposes only and is not legal or career advice. Check your employer's policies and your state's laws to determine what kind of leave you are entitled to.)

Many countries understand that society benefits from helping families off to a healthy start, but unfortunately the US is not one of them. The Family and Medical Leave Act

(FMLA) of 1993 is federal law that requires most, but not all, employers to allow both men and women 12 weeks of parental leave per year. Your employer-provided health insurance has to continue during that time as well. Sounds pretty good, right?

The first problem is that this only means they have to let you come back to work, either to the same position or an equivalent one, after 12 weeks. What they don't have to do is pay you for any part of that 12 weeks.

The second problem is that this only applies to some employers, and to some employees. All public employers, including schools, have to allow parental leave. But private employers only have to comply if they have at least 50 employees.

Then, if your employer is subject to FMLA, the question is do *you* qualify for parental leave. The answer is yes only if you've worked for the employer for at least 12 months (they don't have to be 12 months in a row) and have worked for at least 1,250 hours in the 12 months before your leave starts. Additionally, there must be at least 50 other employees working within 75 miles of where you work.

Keep in mind FMLA is federal law and applies to the bare minimum of what you are entitled to, regardless of where in the US you live. However, you or your employer may be subject to additional state laws, union contracts and other industry-specific requirements. Depending on where you live and what field you work in, you may be entitled to some amount of paid parental leave.

Of course, your employer is free to grant you parental leave if they want to. They can even pay you—if they want to. Some companies do offer paid parental leave as a perk. If your employer, or your partner's employer doesn't, you can always try to negotiate some.

If your job includes paid vacation and sick leave, another

option is to try to save it all up and use it during your leave. If you want to use paid time off to extend your leave beyond 12 weeks you can ask, but your employer doesn't have to agree to it. In some states employers can require you to apply your accrued paid time off to your parental leave.

STRETCHING YOUR PARENTAL LEAVE DOLLAR

STOCKING UP

You may be the exception, but most of us are better at spending money than saving it. This is one time when you can use this to your advantage, though. Rather than trying to put aside money for all the food and other supplies you'll need while one or both of you is on leave, think about what you'll need and buy as much as you can ahead of time. Fill up your garage and closets with all the non-perishable food, paper goods, toiletries, cleaning supplies and baby stuff you're going to need. You may still be broke at the end, but at least you'll have toilet paper.

EQUAL PAY PLANS AND PAYING AHEAD

Do you have heating bills that spike in winter, or cooling bills that explode in summer? Talk to your utility companies about getting on equal payment plans. They will average out your annual costs and break them down into 12 equal payments. Sure, that means you don't get those nice shoulder season months where gas and electric are close to nil, but it's much easier to budget for bills that are the same every month.

Whether you go with an equal payment plan or not, you can pay ahead on utility bills. Calculate how much each will be while you and/or your partner are on leave, and add that amount in when you pay your regular bill. You can do that all at once or pay a little extra each month.

RAINY DAY FUNDS

You've heard that life is what happens while you're busy making other plans. In spite of all your hard work getting ready for this baby, you may find yourself facing expenses you didn't anticipate. It can be difficult, if not impossible, to put money aside when there are already so many financial demands on you.

Brainstorm with your partner and come up with a plan for dealing with financial emergencies. If you can't stuff your mattress with cash, maybe you can have a credit card tucked away that you don't normally use. If you're homeowners, see if you can set up a line of credit on your house.

EDUCATION SAVINGS ACCOUNT

It's never too soon to start saving up for your child's education. In fact, through the magic of compound interest even small amounts paid into a modest interest-bearing savings account will add up substantially over 18 years or so. You have other options, though.

Currently, there are two kinds of educational savings accounts, known as Coverdell Education Savings Accounts (ESAs) and 529 plans. They are different from each other in how you invest your money, and they have different rules on matters such as your income level.

These kind of accounts generally earn a better return on investment than an old school savings account. Even better, as long as you only withdraw the principal and earnings for approved educational purposes, you'll never pay taxes on it.

As with a 401(k), the money is still yours and you can still withdraw it for other purposes, but you'll pay penalties.

The laws on these kind of accounts change from time to time, so you'll need to research current regulations. You might consider talking to an investment or financial counselor.

LIFE INSURANCE

The impending arrival of a new life may not seem like the most likely time to think about death. Part of approaching parenthood as responsible adults, though, is thinking about—and planning for—the unthinkable. It's stressful enough figuring out how to make sure your and your baby's needs are covered with the income or incomes you expect to have. What if something happens to you or your partner and that income disappears?

The answer, of course, is life insurance. It's possible one or both of you already have some through your jobs. Hopefully, you have some kind of disability coverage as well. Check with your employer to see what coverage you have and whether you can or should increase it.

Otherwise, you'll need to think about buying your own insurance. There are a lot of options, so again, you'll need to do some research and get some expert advice.

If one of you will be staying home with the baby and not working for pay, don't make the mistake of thinking you only need to consider insurance for the working partner. The work the stay-at-home partner does also has monetary value, something that becomes crystal clear when you add up what it would cost if you had to hire full-time child and household help.

Certainly the loss of either of you would be catastrophic, and a financial payout wouldn't make that loss any less painful. The point of having life insurance is to make sure whoever is left behind isn't devastated financially as well as emotionally.

WILLS AND ADVANCE DIRECTIVES

On a similar topic, if you and your partner haven't made up wills and advance directives, now is the time.

You and your partner need wills, even if you're not wealthy. Chances are you have something of value to leave behind, whether it's cash, real estate or a comic book collection. A will can cover so much more than dispersal of your worldly goods, though.

If something were to happen to both of you, who would you want to raise your child? If you haven't designated someone in your will, the state will likely take him or her into care and make that decision for you.

What do you want to happen to your social media accounts if you die? Your will can include your user names and passwords, along with instructions on saving your online content and deactivating accounts (or not). If you want to be very thorough you can even leave messages to be posted after your death, although there's a fine line here between being thoughtful and just being creepy.

HEALTH INSURANCE

Ideally, one or both of you will have health insurance that is subsidized by an employer, and that insurance will cover pregnancy and childbirth. Perhaps you have coverage through your state that is based on limited income, or have been able to get coverage on a sliding scale. Otherwise, you may have been paying high premiums for policies that don't cover much, or even going without.

It's best to have health insurance in place before getting pregnant, as whether pregnancy can be considered a preexisting condition for insurance purposes is subject to change. Depending on when and where your partner becomes pregnant, insurers might be able to charge higher premiums or even refuse to insure her.

If you haven't checked your health coverage before now, do it right away. See if your partner is, or can be, added to your policy, or if she has one of her own. Your insurance plan may have a specified open enrollment period during which coverage changes can be made, but pregnancy is usually considered a reason to allow changes outside the enrollment period. Check the pregnancy and childbirth benefits to see what's covered. You'll need to plan for any gaps in coverage.

If your partner doesn't have health insurance and can't find affordable coverage, she may qualify under state-based Medicaid and Children's Health Insurance Program (CHIP). These programs have income requirements and vary from state to state.

Chapter Six
PREPARING YOUR HOME

WHERE WILL THE BABY SLEEP?

It's a very good idea to talk with your partner about where the baby is going to sleep, while keeping in mind that whatever you decide, your feelings may change over time.

Options include a crib, a bassinet, a bassinet attached to your bed, and in the bed with you. Every possibility has its fans and its detractors, and you may be surprised at how strongly some of your friends and family feel about them. The decision about where your baby is going to sleep is deeply personal and should be decided by you and your partner.

If you are setting up a separate room, or nursery, for the baby, you'll have lots of choices as far as materials, colors and lighting.

. . .

CRIB

A crib is the default choice for most parents. A new crib can be expensive and you'll only use it for two or three years at most (less if your child is a precocious climber). You might be offered someone else's old crib or be tempted to buy a used one; if you are, make sure it meets current safety recommendations. Too much space between the bars or between the bottom and side of the crib can trap a baby's body or head, with tragic consequences.

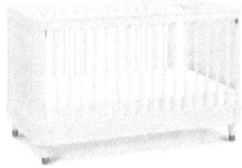

BASSINET

A bassinet is a small cradle-like bed or basket that a baby can sleep in until they are old enough to sit up on their own, around six months or so. At that point the bassinet won't be big enough or stable enough to hold them.

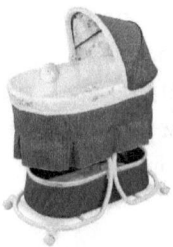

Co-sleeper bassinet

A co-sleeper is a bassinet that fits against the side of your bed. It's a compromise that keeps baby safely in his or her own space, but reassuringly close. It's also possible to "sidecar" a crib by leaving one side off of it and attaching it securely to your bed. Care must be taken to ensure there's no space between bassinet or crib and bed where the baby could get trapped.

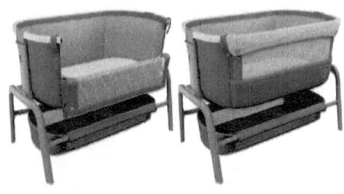

In bed with you

Referred to as co-sleeping or the family bed, keeping your baby in your bed with you may be the most natural option; families have been sleeping together for as long as there have been families. There are many advantages to co-sleeping, and some disadvantages as well. Co-sleeping can enhance bonding with the baby and be especially convenient for breastfeeding; while you won't necessarily get to sleep through the night, you can at least avoid having to get out of bed to attend to diapering or feeding.

On the other hand, co-sleeping may be dangerous for the baby if either you or your partner are big people, heavy sleepers or under the influence of intoxicants or pain medications. And of course, having a baby in the bed changes the dynamic between you and your partner. It's hard to spoon or cuddle with a little body between you. And when you're both ready to start having sex again, a little creativity will be needed if the bed is your usual spot for intimacy.

If you do decide on co-sleeping, it's a good idea to talk about how long you both think you'll want to continue. You may find you love the family bed more than you thought you would, or you may tire of it sooner than expected. And your partner may feel the same—or the opposite! As with so many issues you'll face as parents, it's important to keep the lines of communication open, and to take care of your relationship just as you take care of your child.

HOW MUCH GEAR DO YOU REALLY NEED?

The variety and magnitude of gear for use at home and away is astounding. What you end up with is limited only by your imagination, budget and available space. A reasonable list includes:

Crib, bassinet or other space for baby to sleep.

Blankets. You'll want quite a few of the small, light blankets known commonly called receiving blankets. You'll use them for everything from swaddling the baby to protecting your clothing from spit up. And there will be lots of spit up.

Infant car seat. Most are now designed to accommodate the safety needs of little ones from newborn to toddler. Be wary of used car seats, as it isn't all that uncommon for them to be recalled due to safety issues. Make sure you understand exactly how to secure the seat in your car; practice taking it out and buckling it back in well before your baby is due.

Diapers and wipes or washcloths. Lots of them. You can't even imagine how many diapers you'll go through. There's no doubt disposable diapers are the easiest to deal with, but they do create an enormous landfill burden. Biodegradable diapers are available, but they're not cheap. Cloth diapers can live forever as rags after your baby outgrows them, but they can be a lot of work, and some argue the frequent laundering and disinfection they require isn't a lot greener in the long run. Diaper services that pick up dirty diapers and drop off clean ones may be available.

Seasonally appropriate clothing. Babies aren't very adept at regulating their body temperature for the first year or two. They can easily get overheated if they are overdressed, or become hypothermic if they are underdressed.

Stroller. There are two basic kinds of stroller: the kind that's like a bassinet on wheels, and the kind that is super light and foldable. The first kind lets you carry lots of gear, traverse uneven terrain and protect the baby from sun, wind and rain. The second kind, often called an umbrella stroller, is way less fancy but is easy to pack up and take along. The ideal solution is to have one of each.

MAINTAINING A HEALTHY ENVIRONMENT

DRUGS AND ALCOHOL

Once your baby is crawling, keeping intoxicants out of reach will obviously be an issue. Until then, the concern is passive exposure and the danger of being cared for by adults who are under the influence. Exposing a baby to second hand smoke from pot, crack or meth, or breastfeeding after using any drug, are forms of child abuse, plain and simple. A baby's safety and wellbeing require parents and caregivers to be present, alert and aware of what's happening around them.

· · ·

Tobacco

There's no amount of second-hand tobacco smoke that is safe for a baby. Even limited exposure can contribute to asthma, ear and respiratory infections and even sudden infant death syndrome (SIDS). Smoking inside the home is obviously off limits. Vaping is clearly safer than smoking cigarettes, but that doesn't mean it's safe in your home. You'll still take in toxic amounts of nicotine and other chemicals, and the particulate matter you puff out can still be breathed in by those around you. If either you or your partner is dependent on nicotine in any smoky or vaporous form, now you have a really good reason to quit.

Pets

Besides the emotional benefits of growing up with a beloved pet, research suggests early exposure to furry family members can help prevent a child from developing allergies and asthma. Safety comes first, though. Experts recommend making sure you can control your dog with voice commands, and get it used to baby smells and sounds long before you bring that fragrant little sound machine home. Some dogs will see a newborn as a kind of hairless puppy, while others will see potential prey. Make sure you know which kind of dog you have. The advice for is the same for cats (except for the part about obeying voice commands, of course).

If you have a cat that goes outside and also uses a litter box inside, there are special concerns when your partner is pregnant. If your partner contracts toxoplasmosis while she's pregnant, the parasite can damage the baby's eyes and brain. Toxoplasmosis is a parasite cats pick up by eating infected small animals. The cat then excretes oocysts, which are kind of like tough little eggs, in their feces. Humans become infected by inhaling or swallowing the oocysts. This is obviously a concern with litter boxes, but it can also be a problem if cats use your yard or garden as a toilet. It's best if your partner avoids scooping the litter box while pregnant; if it's unavoidable she should wear gloves and wash her hands afterward.

Chapter Seven

FIRST TRIMESTER - CONCEPTION THROUGH 12 WEEKS

For convenience, pregnancy is divided into trimesters, or three periods each lasting three calendar months. Together they make up the familiar nine-month pregnancy.

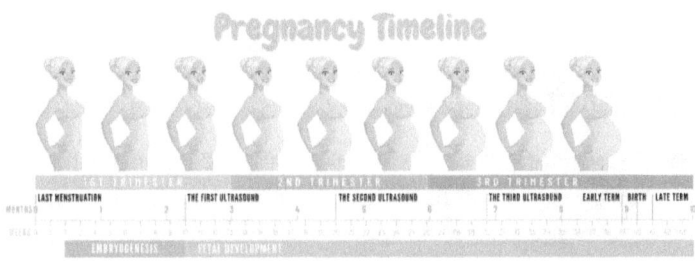

AN OBSTETRICIAN or midwife looks at it a little differently, though. Medically, the average full-term pregnancy lasts 40 weeks. This is counted from the first day of the woman's last menstrual period. If she has a textbook menstrual cycle, she'll have ovulated two weeks after her last period started, and conception will have happened around then. This means that by the time the fertilized egg settles into her uterus, she is already considered to be two weeks pregnant. (Calculations can be more complicated if the egg was fertilized outside your partner's body and implanted into her uterus as an embryo. In this case, your care team will explain how dates will be calculated.)

This calculation helps estimate a due date, or date the baby is expected to be born. The emphasis here is on *expected*—and we know what happens to expectations when it comes to having a baby! The expected due date (EDD) may change as the baby grows and it gets easier to see just how far along it is.

The first trimester can be a little rocky. First there's the joy (or shock) of finding out your partner is pregnant. Then, as her body starts swinging into baby-making mode, the rising tide of hormones makes itself felt. Certain discomforts are very common in the first trimester, and your partner is likely to experience a few.

WHAT THE FIRST TRIMESTER FEELS LIKE

Morning sickness

Most women will have it, but the severity varies. Because hCG, the pregnancy hormone blamed for so many early discomforts, is made by the placenta, morning sickness can be taken as a sign of a healthy placenta that will be part of a healthy pregnancy. Multiple pregnancies (twins, triplets or more) involve multiple placentas, and so morning sickness may be more severe.

Although it tends to be worse in the morning when she wakes up with an empty stomach, morning sickness can occur any time of day. Eating saltine crackers or some similarly bland snack before getting out of bed may help. Ice cubes, popsicles, frequent small meals and ginger supplements or tea throughout the day are other popular treatments.

A less common and more severe form of morning sickness known as hyperemesis gravidarum may require medical care. Hyperemesis means severe vomiting, and it's hard for the woman who suffers it to take in the nutrients she and the baby both need. She may need medication to calm the vomiting, and really bad cases sometimes call for hospitalization. Fortunately, this is rare.

Tender breasts

As much as they are valued for other reasons, breasts are built to feed babies. In the months to come her breasts will get larger and heavier as they get ready for their star turn. Early in pregnancy their heightened state of alert may cause them to become exquisitely tender, especially the nipples. She'll be most comfortable in a close-fitting bra that reduces movement and friction. Don't be surprised to find her wearing one to bed, and don't take it personally if she doesn't want you touching her breasts—at all.

Fatigue

Hormone levels aren't all that's changing in the first trimester. Blood pressure, blood sugar levels and moods may fluctuate as well. Your partner may need more sleep and have less stamina for physical exertion than she normally does. If she has a full-time job she may find it hard to get through her work day and may feel exhausted by the time she gets home.

Remember this is common in the first trimester and she will most likely feel more like herself in a few weeks. Show your support by taking up the slack around the house and encouraging her to rest.

Frequent urination

Later on she'll need to pee a lot because her increased blood volume is kicking her kidneys into overdrive, and because the growing baby is pressing on her bladder. In the first trimester she may feel the need to go a lot because of—you guessed it—hormones.

Sensitivity to tastes and smells

The old TV trope about pregnant women craving pickles and ice cream or some other odd food combination has some basis in fact. She may be repelled by foods she normally loves for reasons she can't really explain, and find that what really hits the spot is something she doesn't usually eat. Overall, of course, the goal is a healthy diet for a healthy pregnancy, but it's fine to indulge her cravings within reason. This is especially true if she also has morning sickness and it's a challenge to get anything down at all.

Headaches

Not every woman will have headaches in the first trimester. For those who do, they may range from mild to migraine. Regular meals and adequate fluids will help prevent headaches caused by low blood sugar or dehydration, although this can be tricky if she has the kind of morning sickness that lasts all day. Headaches can also be a problem if she is trying to cut back on her usual caffeine intake. It's generally a good idea to avoid unnecessary medications in the first trimester when the baby's organs and other parts are forming, but that doesn't mean mom has to suffer. If her headaches are distressing, encourage her to talk to her doctor or midwife about how she can treat them safely.

PRENATAL CARE

Prenatal care covers everything from thinking about getting pregnant to the arrival of the baby. Ideally, your partner will have met with a healthcare provider before getting pregnant, but this may not have happened if she's uninsured or if the pregnancy was a surprise. Otherwise, the first prenatal appointment is usually booked for about eight weeks from the first day of her last period.

If your partner doesn't have health insurance, your local Planned Parenthood clinic is a good place to start looking for prenatal care. She may be able to get all her prenatal care there, either free or at reduced cost. They can also help her find out if she qualifies for health insurance through your state of residence or if there are other affordable health services available.

The first prenatal visit is usually the most comprehensive and will involve a complete health history, physical examination and blood tests. The information gathered will form a baseline that future visits will build on.

After the first visit, a typical timeline for a normal, healthy first pregnancy will include prenatal visits every four weeks for the first 28 weeks, then every two weeks until 36 weeks, and then once a week until the baby comes. Your partner's actual schedule may vary, depending on whether it's her first baby and whether she has, or develops, any health problems.

If it's too early to hear the baby's heartbeat with a handheld Doppler at the first prenatal visit, it will certainly be heard by the second one. First trimester ultrasounds are not routinely done, but may be recommended if a problem is suspected or if it's important to determine just how far along the pregnancy is.

FIRST TRIMESTER SCREEN

Your partner may be offered a combination test known as the first trimester screen. In the first part of the test, her blood is tested for substances that might indicate the baby has Down syndrome or certain other uncommon chromosomal abnormalities. The second part of the test is an ultrasound that measures tissue at the back of the baby's neck. Taken together, these two tests make it possible to estimate the *risk* of an abnormality, not the presence of an abnormality. If the screen suggests there is a medium to high risk, more testing can be done.

THE AWKWARD BITS

VAGINAL ODOR

Changes in hormone levels and vaginal pH may cause your partner's odor to be stronger, or just different, than usual. It may even smell something like what she had to eat for lunch. This is perfectly normal. A strong fishy odor though, may be a symptom of a bacterial infection that needs attention. You can try to find a gentle way to alert your partner if you think her smell is abnormal, but with her increased sensitivity to odors she probably already knows.

GAS AND CONSTIPATION

The hormones of pregnancy tend to cause muscles to relax. The GI system relies on muscular contractions to keep food moving as it's digested, and it can slow down a bit in pregnancy. The result is often constipation, bloating and gassiness. Gas is released as bacteria in the intestines break down nutrients, so the longer it takes for the nutrients to move through, the more gas can be produced. The anus is, of course, part of the GI system, and holding in gas requires a tightening of anal muscles. As those muscles soften, your partner may be dismayed to discover her farts taking on a life of their own, popping out at the most inopportune moments. Do your best to laugh with her, not at her.

STRESS INCONTINENCE

In the last trimester, especially, the weight of the growing baby will press against your partner's bladder. Not only will she need to pee a lot, she may find that anything that increases pressure in her abdomen—like sneezing, for example—may cause urine to leak right out. This is called stress incontinence. If this happens to her she might want to wear panty liners.

FACIAL HAIR

Your partner may find something growing in pregnancy she definitely didn't count on: a beard. In fact, she may notice new hair on other parts of her body as well, including on her belly and around her nipples. This is partly due to new hair growth, partly to hair growing in a bit darker than usual, and partly to hairs not falling out as they normally would. All of this is perfectly normal and temporary.

HEMORRHOIDS

Hemorrhoids are swollen veins in the rectum and around the anus. They are a very common discomfort of pregnancy.

Early on they may be caused by constipation, and later by the increased pressure of an abdomen full of baby. They may also result from, or be made worse by, the strain of pushing the baby out. The best defense against hemorrhoids is to prevent constipation by taking in lots of fiber and fluids, getting regular exercise and going to the bathroom as soon as the need arises (rather than holding it for a more convenient time).

Leaking breasts

Long before the baby comes, your partner's breasts may begin producing a thick, creamy fluid called colostrum. It will take a few days after the baby is born for her breasts to fill with milk, and the colostrum will tide the baby over until they do. Not every woman will leak like this during pregnancy. If your partner does, she may want to wear breast pads, or nursing pads, inside her bra. They will come in handy after the baby comes, too, as it isn't uncommon for a nursing mother's breasts to leak milk when they're full or even when she hears a baby cry.

Chapter Eight
SECOND TRIMESTER - 13 TO 27 WEEKS

For many women, the second trimester is the most enjoyable part of pregnancy. Morning sickness resolves, her energy returns, she starts feeling the baby move and everything seems to be falling into place. Or not.

PHYSICAL CHANGES

The second trimester is when your partner is likely to start really looking and feeling pregnant. Her growing bump is not the only noticeable change, though. While every woman is an individual and every pregnancy is unique, there are some features that are common to this stage.

Melasma

Melanin is the brown pigment that determines skin color. Exposure to the sun causes an increase in melanin, but pregnancy hormones can stimulate melanin production too. Melasma is sometimes called the "mask of pregnancy" because it is seen so commonly on the faces of pregnant women. It shows up even on women whose skin is naturally rich in melanin. The downside of melasma is that it tends to be patchy and uneven. The good news is that it should fully resolve after the baby comes. In the meantime, your partner should be sure to use a good, broad-spectrum sunscreen with an SPF of at least 30 whenever she's in the sun.ù

Linea negra

This is a dark line, sometimes called the pregnancy line, on a pregnant woman's abdomen that runs from the belly button down to the pubic bone. Sometimes it extends above the belly button to the ribs. It's another instance of increased melanin production that usually resolves after the baby is born, although it may take a few months to disappear completely.

Stretch marks

Whether your partner gets stretch marks, and how pronounced they are, depends partly on genetics and partly on how much weight she gains, and how quickly. They may develop on her belly, breasts, thighs or buttocks and are due to tearing of connective tissue under the skin. Stretch marks usually look red or purple during pregnancy and fade in color afterward, although they never actually go away. The stretching skin over her belly is likely to be itchy, too. Although there's no science behind claims that coconut butter or other salves will prevent stretch marks, keeping the skin well-moisturized may help with the itching.

Braxton Hicks contractions

These "practice" contractions usually kick in during the

second trimester, becoming more intense in the third. Your partner will notice her belly becoming tighter and then relaxing, occasionally at first and more frequently as time goes on. It's possible she will find them startling or uncomfortable; some women like to visualize them as giving the baby a big hug. Braxton Hicks contractions don't open the cervix and are not a sign of early labor, but your partner should definitely check in with her doctor or midwife if she's worried.

Round ligament pain

As her belly grows and gets heavier, your partner may sometimes have sharp pains in her groin, usually to one side or the other (or both), rather than in the middle. The pain is due to pressure on, and spasming of, the round ligaments that support the uterus. She may experience stabbing pains when she changes position suddenly, such as when rolling over and sitting up in bed, or when coughing or sneezing. She may not be able to avoid round ligament pain altogether, but changing position more slowly and gently may help.

Fetal movement

Some time during the second trimester, your partner will start feeling the baby move. The first time may be sudden, like it is on TV. It is more likely, though, that she will gradually become aware that what she thought were just more gas bubbles moving through her intestines are actually kicks and pokes from her little passenger. Traditionally the onset of noticeable fetal movement was known as "quickening"—ie, the beginning of life.

People often refer to fetal movement as "kicking" but the baby does much more than kick in there. As it grows it will sometimes feel like it's doing tai kwon do, and it will in fact do gymnastics, including somersaults. In time you'll be able to feel the movements by putting your hand on her belly, and eventually you'll be able to see them. You may even get to where you can confidently identify a moving part as a foot or an elbow!

Libido

First trimester discomforts may have resolved, but hormones are still running high. Your partner may feel very sexy, the most extreme opposite of sexy, or something in between. Creating life is probably the most intimate thing two people can do together, and you may find your lovemaking increasingly tender and loving. If you're not on the same page sexually, though, there's plenty of opportunity for conflict and resentment. Maybe you find her more beautiful and desirable than ever, but she pushes you away. Maybe her libido is at a peak but you can't help feeling weird about having sex with a baby onboard. This is another opportunity to practice the open, honest communication that will help get you through the coming challenges of parenthood.

PRENATAL CARE

During the second trimester your partner will probably see her healthcare provider about every four weeks.

Fundal height

During these visits the healthcare provider will measure the distance from your partner's pubic bone to the top of her uterus, known as the fundal height. This is done to estimate the baby's size and how it compares to how far along in pregnancy your partner is thought to be.

After 20 weeks the fundal height in centimeters is expected to match the number of weeks of pregnancy, so for example at 25 weeks the fundal height should be 25 centimeters. Fundal height is a convenient guide to fetal growth but not always 100 percent accurate. If there are any concerns about the baby's size or whether the due date has been estimated correctly, an ultrasound will probably be ordered.

Fetal heartbeat

Listening to the baby's heartbeat with the handheld Doppler is often the highlight of second trimester visits, even if you've heard it before. It's reassurance that your baby is doing well and may help you, the dad, feel more connected to him or her.

Ultrasound

While they aren't really necessary for normal pregnancies, ultrasounds have become very common. If your partner hasn't already had one it's likely one it's likely to be offered now, and that peek into the baby's hidden world is hard to resist. It may be possible to determine the gender by this point, so you should decide beforehand whether or not you want to know. Ultrasounds can be hard to decipher and it's possible only the technician will be able to tell for sure, but sometimes it's pretty obvious, especially if you get a 3D ultrasound. Of course, the medical rationale for ultrasound is to make sure everything is okay, and so measurements will be taken and limbs and organs will be inspected to make sure there aren't any obvious problems.

Urine test

On each prenatal visit, your partner will be asked to provide a urine sample to check for gestational diabetes (sugar in the urine), preeclampsia (protein in the urine) and urinary tract infection (white blood cells in the urine). This is usually done by dipping a testing strip into the sample, and in some offices your partner will be able to do this herself.

Weight

Your partner's weight will be checked at every visit to make sure she's gaining at a healthy rate. If she was underweight or had a healthy BMI when she got pregnant, she'll be expected to gain about a pound a week during the second trimester. Some of this is the baby, but most of it is a combination of body fat, amniotic fluid and increased blood volume. If she started out with a high BMI, her goal will be to gain about half a pound per week.

Genetic testing

Testing for genetic abnormalities may be offered during the second trimester, especially if either you or your partner are known to carry a genetic condition, or if there are any conditions that run in either of your families. A quad test, or quad marker screen, checks for substances in your partner's blood that might indicate the baby has problems with the brain or spinal cord, or has Down syndrome or another chromosomal abnormality. Like the first trimester screen, the quad test measures *risk* of abnormality, not the presence of abnormality. A calculated risk that is medium or high can be confirmed with ultrasound and amniocentesis.

Amniocentesis

Amniocentesis involves inserting a needle into the uterus and withdrawing some of the amniotic fluid the baby is floating in. Genetic testing can be done on cells from the baby that are found in the amniotic fluid. Amniocentesis is highly accurate and can screen for a number of conditions that can't be diagnosed before birth by any other means. It does carry a small risk of miscarriage, though, and an even smaller risk of infection or early labor.

Amniocentesis is strictly optional, and if it's offered or recommended you and your partner will need to weigh the risks and benefits before deciding if you want to go through with it. Knowing about a problem can give you time to get ready for a baby that will have special needs, or to consider terminating the pregnancy if the problems are very severe.

Chapter Nine

THIRD TRIMESTER - 28 TO 40 WEEKS

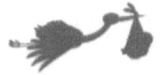

The third trimester is when pregnancy, and the fact that a baby is on the way, becomes obvious and real. The seventh month is when your partner's bump blossoms, especially if this is her first baby. It may be hard to believe it's going to get even bigger over the next two months!

After feeling cheerful and energetic during the second trimester, she may now start slowing down and facing some new discomforts. All of this is balanced, of course, with the excitement and anticipation of the baby's arrival—the big payoff for all this hard work.

By 28 weeks the baby's parts are all built and refined, and now all that's left is to grow, fill out and generally get ready for life outside the womb. This can be a joyous and busy time for you and your partner, and a time that brings its own challenges.

THE BABY BUMP

Up until now, the changes in your partner's body may have been somewhat subtle. Yes, her belly rounded and she may have added some extra padding elsewhere, but the changes might not have been pregnancy-specific. From here on out, they will be much more so.

The size, weight and shape of her belly will begin to change her center of gravity. Ligaments in her pelvis are also softening and loosening, and she may start to walk and move very differently.

If you have access to an empathy or sympathy belly, it will help give you some insight into what your partner is experiencing. An empathy belly is a weighted vest that gives you an idea of what it feels like to carry the size and weight of a pregnant belly and breasts. You may not be likely to have one lying around, but you'll probably get a chance to try one out in your childbirth preparation classes.

Belly bands and support belts

The female pelvis is wider than the male pelvis, with a larger opening in the center, perfect for passing a baby through. Except, have you seen the size of a newborn baby? Have you ever looked at your partner and wondered how on earth that's going to work?

Part of the answer lies in the changes that take place in the pelvis in the last trimester. The pelvis isn't just one solid piece; it has joints, and ligaments holding the joints together. In pregnancy the ligaments get looser, allowing some remodeling of the pelvis. This is good news when it's time to birth that baby, but in the meantime it can cause some discomfort.

The pressure of the baby on stretched ligaments can cause pain in the pelvis, groin and back. One way to help ease this discomfort is to wear a belly band or maternity support belt. There are many different designs, but they are kind of first cousins to the support belts worn for hernias and heavy lifting. Basically, a belly band or belt goes around the back and under the belly, supporting it and relieving ligament strain.

SLEEPING POSITION

Your partner may have been advised not to sleep on her back during the last trimester. This is because the weight of the baby can compress the vena cava, a large blood vessel that runs under the uterus. Squeezing the vena cava can cause her blood pressure to drop. In theory, this low blood pressure can cause her to feel dizzy and nauseated and possibly deprive the baby of needed oxygen. The science doesn't really back this up, though, and if your partner finds she only sleeps well on her back she probably doesn't need to worry about it. She can always clear it with her doctor or midwife, just to be sure. It's also possible that she'll find sleeping on her back impossible anyway, as pressure on her diaphragm can make it hard to breathe. She may sleep much better on her side, especially with lots of pillows to tuck around her belly and between her legs.

PREGNANCY BRAIN

Yes, this is a real thing. Feeling spacey and forgetful in the third trimester is reassuringly common. Your partner may need lots of notes and lists to help navigate her daily life, whether it's reminding her of an appointment she has made, or even why she walked into that room. This is due in part to hormones, of course—isn't everything at this point?—but there are other factors at play as well. Her growing belly, weird dreams and need to pee during the night may be causing some sleep deprivation. Having so much to do before the baby arrives may be stressing her out, and stress makes everyone forgetful. And finally, she is likely becoming preoccupied with thoughts of childbirth and caring for a newborn. One theory is that losing focus on other things and thinking more about the baby is just what nature intends. In any case, pregnancy brain is a temporary disability.

INCREASED BLOOD VOLUME

To meet the demands of building a new human, your partner's total blood volume has by now increased by 50 percent, or about 1250 ml. That's 42 ounces, or more than five cups. This is great for the baby, but all that extra fluid can have some unpleasant side effects for mom. She may notice swelling of her fingers, toes, feet and ankles. She may develop varicose veins in her legs, and her nose may feel stuffy. And of course there's the frequent need to pee, which is partially due to the baby sitting on her bladder but also to her kidneys processing all that extra fluid. She should talk with her doctor or midwife about appropriate comfort measures and treatment options, which may include support stockings, salt water nasal rinses, elevating her feet and removing jewelry, especially rings.

ACTIVITY

Many women stay very active right up until they go into labor, whether because they want to or because they have no choice—the world doesn't stop and wait for your baby to come, after all. If your partner was athletic before getting pregnant and hasn't faced any unexpected complications, she may keep up her usual pace and feel quite comfortable doing so. Even so, no woman completely escapes the physical reality of late pregnancy.

Kick counting

By the third trimester your partner should be feeling the baby move quite regularly. By 30 weeks she'll want to start paying attention to just how often she feels movement. In addition to her general awareness of the baby's activity, she may be advised to have a couple of times each day when she actually counts how many times in an hour the baby moves.

We tend to talk about the baby "kicking," and sometimes it does feel like feet are flying, but that's not all that's going on. Most babies don't settle into one position until just before labor begins; until then, they move in every direction and at any given moment may be upside down, right side up or lying sideways. They may face outward, toward mom's spine or off to the side.

Whatever is going on in there, some kind of activity should be felt at least six times per hour. Your partner will likely be advised to set aside a couple of times each day for kick counting, in which she should sit quietly and count the number of movements she feels. Babies in the womb do sleep and will have quiet times, but your partner should check in with her doctor or midwife if she's feeling less movement than expected.

PHYSICAL PREPARATION

A baby carried to term is going to be born one way or another, whether you and your partner prepare or not. If she's planning to deliver vaginally (the old school way), though, there are some things she can do to get in shape for the big event. There's even something you can help with.

. . .

KEGEL EXERCISES

Kegels can be tedious, but doing them doesn't just help your partner prepare for childbirth; it also helps her get back into shape afterward. Kegels work the pelvic floor muscles that support the uterus, bladder and intestines. Keeping these muscles strong will help her do the hard work of childbirth and also help her bounce back afterward.

Men also have pelvic floor muscles, and doing Kegels can help treat and prevent dribbling and erectile dysfunction. Kegel time can be couple time!

To activate the right muscles, pretend you are trying to hold in urine or gas. Squeeze for a count of five and release. Three sets of 10 reps per day is ideal, both for you and for your partner.

PERINEAL MASSAGE

The perineum is the space between the vagina and the anus (or in your case, between the scrotum and the anus). Women are often advised to spend some time massaging and stretching their perineum before giving birth for the first time. The hope is that this will help keep the perineum, which can tear or be cut to make more room for the baby to emerge, intact. Studies haven't found really strong evidence perineal massage works, but it can't hurt.

It's generally recommended to place two lubricated fingers part way into the vagina and apply firm but gentle pressure, first downward toward the anus and then to each side. It's easier for you to do this than for your partner to do it for herself, especially late in pregnancy when she may have trouble reaching that far at all. She should check with her doctor or midwife first to make sure there's no reason she should avoid perineal massage.

CHILDBIRTH PREPARATION CLASSES

Childbirth classes are usually planned to begin around six or seven months into pregnancy. They can be scheduled later, but there's always the chance your baby will surprise you with an early appearance, leaving you unprepared.

Traditionally, classes are offered through, and usually at, the facility where you're planning to have the baby. If that's a hospital or birthing center, classes are likely to include a tour of the labor and delivery areas. If you're planning a home birth, classes may be offered with a midwife, birth assistant or doula, and the location will vary.

Nowadays there are many ways to approach childbirth preparation. Many of the places that offer classes in a series also offer "express" preparation that fits everything into one class. And of course there are video and live-streamed online classes.

Classes can include everything from fetal development to childbirth to newborn care, or can be broken down into separate classes for each topic. They may focus on one particular approach to childbirth, such as Lamaze or the Bradley method, or they may touch on aspects of many.

The kind of preparation you and your partner choose will depend on your previous experience and knowledge base, your schedules and learning styles, and the kind of birth you hope to have.

MAKING A BIRTH PLAN

A birth plan is the very epitome of hoping for the best and planning for the worst. You and your partner should think about how you want the delivery to go, and also how you want to respond if things don't go according to plan. You should write your plan out, give a copy to the doctor or midwife and to the birth assistant or doula if you have one, and pack a copy in with your birth kit or go bag.

You can get a birth plan template from a healthcare provider or find one online. You can make it as simple or as comprehensive as you like, covering everything from whether your partner wants an epidural to what music she wants to have playing while she's in labor to whether you will allow the baby to be bathed.

Just keep in mind that circumstances may not allow everything to play out the way you plan, and your partner may change her mind as labor progresses. She might find she wants a different playlist (or no music at all), or be surprised by which comfort measures actually help the most. If she wants to avoid an epidural or other pain medication, she needs to think about how important this is to her—if she finds herself wanting something for pain after all, does she want you to agree, or try to talk her out of it?

Just keep in mind a birth plan is more of a wish list than a recipe. Surprises, whether large or small, are inevitable.

WHAT THE BABY'S DOING

THE BABY DROPS

The ideal position for a baby to be in before labor begins is head down, facing mom's spine. There's some maneuvering to be done when it's time to slip under the public bone on the way to the birth canal, and being oriented this way is best. At some point before labor begins, either just before or even weeks before, most babies will drop lower into mom's pelvis and settle into this head-down position. Less commonly a baby settles in right side up, or breech.

A traditional term for this settling is lightening, because the woman often feels much lighter in her upper abdomen as space increases for her stomach and diaphragm. She may breathe easier and have relief from indigestion and heartburn. At the same time, though, she may feel much more pressure lower down, aggravating hemorrhoids, decreasing her bladder capacity and sometimes even making walking awkward. This change in the baby's position is also known as dropping or engaging.

Chapter Ten

COMPLICATIONS IN PREGNANCY

The best defense against complications in pregnancy is a healthy lifestyle and good prenatal care. But complications can arise, and may be due to factors completely out of your and your partner's control.

Some of these complications are pretty scary. It's good to be aware of symptoms that need attention, but also to remember you probably won't be dealing with any of the really serious ones.

MISCARRIAGE

One or two out of every 10 confirmed pregnancies will end in miscarriage, usually within the first trimester. It's something to be aware of, but not to spend a lot of time worrying about. Remember, this means eight to nine out of every 10 confirmed pregnancies carry on and result in a baby.

In most cases, the reason for an early miscarriage is never known. It will usually be assumed there was a problem with that particular pregnancy that kept it from developing further. For most women, miscarriage is a one-off. It may cause some anxiety the next time around, but it's overwhelmingly likely it won't happen again.

A very small number of women do go on to have a second or even a third early pregnancy loss. This is known as recurrent miscarriage. After a third miscarriage, an investigation into what's causing this to happen is likely to be done. A cause isn't always found, though, and even women who have had recurrent miscarriages more often than not go on to have successful pregnancies.

Symptoms

Miscarriage sometimes happens in real life the way it does on TV, but usually it does not. Rather than a dramatic event with sudden severe pain and heavy bleeding, the end of an early pregnancy is likely to sneak up on you. In fact, the first sign of an impending miscarriage may be that your partner suddenly feels much better. As hormone levels fall she may celebrate the end of morning sickness and the other early discomforts. Later, cramping and spotting make it clear the pregnancy is in trouble.

At this point she will most likely be sent in for an ultrasound to determine "fetal viability," that is, whether or not the fetus is still alive. If it is not, decisions will need to be made about how to proceed.

In most cases, she will be sent home, possibly with something to take for pain. Depending on how far along she was, she may experience something like a normal or severe period, or even something more like labor pains, because her cervix must dilate to allow the uterine contents to pass. This may take hours or days. She may pass blood clots and indistinct tissue, or even a recognizable fetus. If that happens, you'll need to think about what you want to do with the remains.

How to say goodbye to a much hoped-for baby is a very personal decision.

Complications

Bleeding may continue for a few days, much like a regular period. Heavy bleeding, bleeding for more than a few days, foul-smelling discharge, fever or flu-like symptoms require medical care. It isn't common but sometimes tissue remains in the uterus, leading to what is known as an incomplete miscarriage. This can cause heavy bleeding and infection, and sometimes a procedure is needed to remove what's been left behind.

ECTOPIC PREGNANCY

Conception—the meeting of the egg and the sperm—takes place in the fallopian tubes, the very narrow channels eggs pass through when they leave the ovaries. In a normal pregnancy, the fertilized egg continues along until it reaches the uterus and settles in.

In an ectopic pregnancy, the egg settles in somewhere other than the uterus, usually the fallopian tube itself. Less common spots include the ovary and the cervix. Because there's a tiny space between the fallopian tubes and the ovaries, in very rare cases a fertilized egg may escape the reproductive system altogether and travel out into the abdomen.

An ectopic pregnancy is not a normal pregnancy, and a woman who has one may or may not have typical symptoms of early pregnancy. Whether she feels pregnant or not, at some point she will start noticing pain in her pelvis that is definitely different from menstrual cramps, and she may have some vaginal bleeding.

An ectopic pregnancy in a fallopian tube, also known as a tubal pregnancy, may grow large enough to rupture the tube, causing severe pain and bleeding. Sometimes an ectopic pregnancy bleeds internally. When this happens, she may feel intense pressure in her rectum and lower abdomen, have shooting pain up into her back and shoulders and feel dizzy and lightheaded. A ruptured ectopic pregnancy is a medical emergency and can be life-threatening.

There is no way to save an ectopic pregnancy, and it can never result in a baby. Once your partner is out of physical danger, grieving over the loss of the pregnancy is likely to begin. If the fallopian tube was damaged beyond repair it will be harder to conceive again, and this may add to the emotional toll.

HYDATIFORM MOLE

It is very unlikely your partner will have a hydatiform mole, also known as molar pregnancy, as they are pretty rare. Like an ectopic pregnancy, a molar pregnancy will not result in a baby.

A hydatiform mole grows from tissue that would form the placenta in a normal pregnancy. In a complete molar pregnancy, an egg is fertilized by the father's sperm but for some reason the mother's share of DNA is missing. In a partial molar pregnancy, the mother's DNA is present but there are two copies of the father's DNA, possibly because the egg has been fertilized by two sperm.

In a complete molar pregnancy no embryo is formed at all. In a partial molar pregnancy the embryo may begin to form but won't be viable and will eventually miscarry. In rare cases a molar pregnancy may grow from tissue left behind after a miscarriage or normal delivery. Even more rarely, a molar pregnancy can turn cancerous.

A molar pregnancy may start out just like a normal pregnancy, but usually grows much faster. Instead of a slow-growing baby bump, a woman may suddenly look very pregnant very early on. She is likely to have bleeding and severe morning sickness as well. A molar pregnancy is an uncommon but serious complication that requires immediate medical attention.

HYPEREMESIS GRAVIDARUM

More than just severe morning sickness, hyperemesis gravidarum is severe nausea and vomiting in pregnancy that causes weight loss, dehydration and electrolyte imbalances. It can make it impossible for the woman to take in the nutrients she and the baby need, and can affect her kidneys, liver and thyroid function.

Sometimes hyperemesis can be managed with comfort measures at home. Sometimes IV fluids are needed to replace body fluids lost through vomiting and being unable to drink water. In extreme cases, a woman may have to be hospitalized and liquid nutrition delivered through an IV or stomach tube. As a last resort the pregnancy may have to be terminated.

GESTATIONAL DIABETES

You may be familiar with diabetes. Type I is the kind where your pancreas doesn't produce enough insulin. Insulin is needed to move glucose, or sugar, from the blood into cells, where it's used for energy. Without insulin, glucose builds up in the blood and cells are starved for energy. A person with Type I diabetes has to inject insulin.

Type II diabetes, which is becoming increasingly common in the US, is the kind where you produce insulin but your cells don't respond to it properly. Type II diabetes can often be reversed with lifestyle changes.

Gestational diabetes only occurs during pregnancy. It develops in the third trimester and doesn't usually cause any noticeable symptoms, so your partner will be tested for it at a prenatal visit between 24 and 28 weeks. It's believed that in gestational diabetes, hormones from the placenta keep the woman from producing as much insulin she needs or from being able to use the insulin she does produce.

The growing baby is the loser in this tug-of-war between insulin and blood sugar. Insulin doesn't cross the placenta but glucose does, putting the baby in danger of developing high blood sugar, or hyperglycemia, in the uterus. This can cause problems for the baby both before and after birth.

Gestational diabetes can usually be managed with exercise, a healthy diet and careful monitoring of blood sugar levels. Sometimes, though, a woman may temporarily need insulin.

Gestational diabetes should resolve once the baby is born, but there is a risk the woman will go on to develop Type II diabetes afterward. If your partner develops gestational diabetes, her blood sugar will be monitored after the baby comes to make sure it returns to normal.

GESTATIONAL HYPERTENSION

Some women with normal blood pressure (120/80 or less) will develop high blood pressure (140/90 or higher) while pregnant, usually around 20 weeks. Sometimes it gets high enough to be worrisome, but it usually doesn't cause any problems and goes back to normal after the baby is born. It does increase the possibility the woman will develop chronic hypertension in the future, though.

PREECLAMPSIA

When a pregnant woman develops high blood pressure and signs of injury to vital organs like her kidneys or liver, this is called preeclampsia. Preeclampsia is very serious and has to be managed carefully to keep it from becoming life-threatening. Whereas gestational hypertension tends not to have any symptoms, preeclampsia can cause headaches, vision problems, abdominal pain, trouble breathing and swelling of the hands and face. Symptoms like these indicate preeclampsia is developing and urgent medical care is needed.

If your partner becomes preeclamptic she may be admitted to the hospital for treatment. The only cure for preeclampsia is to deliver the baby, so if she is at least 37 weeks along this will be strongly recommended. If she isn't yet at 37 weeks every effort will be made to keep her condition under control until she gets there, but if it can't be controlled the baby will need to be delivered anyway.

PROBLEMS WITH THE PLACENTA

The two main problems that can develop with the placenta are called placenta previa and placenta abruption.

Until the baby is born and begins breathing on its own, it is completely dependent on the placenta for its oxygen. The placenta remains attached to the uterus throughout labor and birth, absorbing oxygen from mom's blood and passing it to the baby through the umbilical cord. If the placenta separates from the uterus before the baby is born, the effects can be catastrophic.

A previa is when the placenta attaches very low in the uterus, partly or completely covering the cervix. Sometimes, as the baby grows and the uterus expands, the placenta will be pulled up away from the cervix. If this doesn't happen the baby will have to be delivered by cesarean section.

An abruption is when the placenta pulls away from the uterine wall before the baby is born. This can happen slowly or all at once. If it happens slowly over the course of the pregnancy the baby may be deprived of oxygen and nutrients. If it happens suddenly the baby can die. The heavy bleeding from a sudden abruption can be life-threatening for the mother as well.

POSTDATES/OVERDUE

When your partner first found out she was pregnant, her estimated due date (EDD) was calculated by adding 280 days to the first day of her last period. That works out to a little over nine months, or 40 weeks to be more exact. At each of her prenatal appointments and during any ultrasounds she has, the baby is measured, its state of development is determined and the EDD adjusted accordingly.

A full-term pregnancy has been defined in different ways through the years, but that 40-week standard has stuck. Generally, a baby born between about 39 and 41 weeks is considered full-term. Earlier than 39 weeks is early, and more than 41 weeks is late. These are just guidelines, however, as perfectly healthy babies may be born at 38 or 42 weeks.

If labor hasn't started by 42 weeks at the latest, though, medical intervention will be strongly advised. A baby who stays in the womb longer than this may grow so big it's hard to deliver. It may also suffer as the placenta starts to deteriorate and the amount of amniotic fluid drops. There's also an increased risk of stillbirth.

You can be sure that by 40 weeks your partner will be done with being pregnant and will want very much for the baby to come. Some women find walking as much as possible helps. If the baby hasn't settled into a good position for birth it may be possible to use gravity and body movements to persuade it to do so. Certain herbal teas or extracts are sometimes suggested. Nipple stimulation and orgasm are often recommended to get the uterus contracting. Your partner should check in with her doctor or midwife before trying any of these.

MEDICAL INTERVENTIONS TO GET LABOR STARTED

RIPENING THE CERVIX

The primary measure of how well labor is progressing is the dilation and effacement, or opening and thinning, of the cervix. There are a number of different substances that can be applied directly to the cervix to "ripen" it, or cause it to soften. Sometimes ripening the cervix is enough to get labor started. Otherwise, it's done to prepare the cervix before induction, because the closer to ready the cervix is, the more likely induction will be successful.

AMNIOTOMY

The amniotic sac in which the baby floats in its amniotic fluid nearly always ruptures before birth, although rarely in a sudden, dramatic cascade as it does on TV. If your partner's cervix has thinned out and started to dilate and the baby's head is pressing on it—basically, at the starting gate, waiting for the race to begin—the doctor or midwife might go ahead and rupture the membranes. When the rupture is intentional it's called an amniotomy. In many cases this will jump start contractions and get labor going. Once the membranes have ruptured, though, whether naturally or through amniotomy, the clock starts ticking, as the baby is now unprotected from infection that could reach it through the vagina. If amniotomy doesn't work to get labor started, the next step is induction or C-section.

Induction

If your partner hasn't gone into labor naturally by 41 or 42 weeks, and if the baby looks healthy and like it will still fit through the birth canal, labor may be induced.

This is done in the hospital, by infusing Pitocin intravenously. Pitocin is a synthetic form of oxytocin, the hormone responsible for uterine contractions. It has a bad reputation for causing severely painful contractions, but managed properly it can bring on contractions that slowly increase in intensity just like they naturally would.

The benefit of getting labor started with Pitocin has to be weighed against the risks, which include causing stress on the baby. If your partner has had a C-section previously, strong Pitocin contractions increase the risk of the uterus rupturing along the old incision. And not every Pitocin induction is successful; if labor still doesn't progress, a C-section could still be necessary.

Chapter Eleven

GOING INTO LABOR

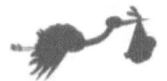

So this is how it works: you and your partner are going about your normal business, maybe having a nice dinner, when suddenly she grabs her belly and gasps, "Honey, it's time!" Maybe her water breaks first, flooding the floor beneath her, and with wide eyes she exclaims, "The baby is coming!" Then you jump in the car or taxi, possibly leaving her behind in your haste, and race to the hospital. Hopefully you get there in time and she makes it to a bed before she starts sweating and screaming at the top of her lungs and the baby comes shooting out.

Right?

LOL. Forget everything you think you know about labor and childbirth from TV and movies. There is such a thing as precipitous labor that is short and sweet, but that's extremely rare. For most women, especially first-time moms, the reality is much, much different.

For one thing, her labor is very unlikely to start suddenly and obviously. The segue from Braxton Hicks "practice" contractions to "real" labor contractions can be very subtle. It may take hours or even days for your partner to be sure something different is going on. Even then, it probably isn't time to race off to the hospital.

Here's a quick timeline of the labor stages. Later, we'll talk more about the actual birth.

STAGES OF LABOR

The uterus is a muscular organ. In labor the uterus contracts, pulling the cervix open and pushing the baby down and out. How long labor and each of its stages lasts is variable. For a first-time mom, there's usually at least 24 hours between the time she realizes she's in labor and the birth of the baby.

FIRST STAGE

The first stage of labor is when the cervix opens, or dilates, and thins out, or effaces. It's broken down into three phases of its own that are defined by what's going on with the cervix.

PHASE ONE: EARLY LABOR

Phase one goes until the cervix has dilated 3 cm, roughly the size of a quarter. Some women will have already dilated to 1 cm weeks before labor starts. During this phase contractions are noticeable but tend to be irregular and relatively mild. Your partner may feel like she has menstrual cramps, and she may feel the contractions in her back. They last about 30 to 45 seconds, with anywhere from 5 to 30 minute in between. It's hard to say how long this phase will take—it could be days. Your partner will stay in touch with her doctor or midwife during early labor but most likely will stay at home.

. . .

Phase two: Active labor

During active labor the cervix dilates to 7 cm, about the diameter of a peach. Contractions get longer, stronger and closer together, lasting 45 to 60 seconds with about three to five minutes in between. If your partner is delivering at a hospital or birth center, this is the time to go there—safely, not in a panic. If you're having a home birth the midwife and doula or birth assistant will be in attendance.

Phase three: Transition

This is the part where women on TV grab their partners by the collar and curse at them. As her cervix approaches 10 cm dilation, about the diameter of a grapefruit, your partner could become quite emotional—don't take any outbursts personally. She may already be feeling the urge to push, but she'll have to fight that urge until the cervix is fully open. Starting to push before the cervix is ready can cause it to swell so that it not only stops opening, it actually closes some. You will have learned some techniques in your childbirth preparation classes to help her through this phase, so use them!

Second stage

This is it! The second stage is when her cervix is fully dilated and your partner can begin pushing. As with the other stages, it's hard to say how long this one will last, but as with the others it's usually longer for a first-time mom. Minutes or hours, this stage is hard work and can be grueling. With the finish line in sight your partner may be energized and determined, but if it takes a while she can become exhausted and discouraged. She will need your support now more than ever.

Once the baby is born it will be quickly examined to make

sure there are no problems, the cord will be cut, and it will be placed on mom's chest so the three of you can start bonding and getting acquainted. However, if the baby needs any kind of special care it may be taken out of the room and the bonding will have to wait.

Third stage

The delivery of the placenta is the least-glamorous stage of labor, but it still requires the careful attention of the doctor or midwife. They will examine the placenta carefully to make sure it's intact. Any pieces left behind can interfere with the uterus contracting back to its normal size, and that can cause serious bleeding. Fortunately, this is not at all common. It is more likely the placenta will be whole and everything will proceed normally.

When making your birth plan you and your partner probably discussed what, if anything, you wanted to do with the placenta. Some couples will take theirs home and use it to nourish a tree they plant in honor of their child's birth. There are those who advocate eating the placenta, something other mammals do, although there's no scientific basis for claims about its nutritional value. You and your partner may not really care what happens to the placenta, and that's fine, too. Leave it behind and it will be disposed of properly.

Chapter Twelve

WHO'S GOING TO BE THERE WHEN THE BABY COMES?

*J*ust as there are many ways to give birth, there are many kinds of healthcare practitioners who may be involved. Your individual cast of characters may end up including only those you know and expect, or there may stand-ins, understudies or unexpected walk-ons. It's good to know who might be there.

If you are having multiples or if there are other special circumstances, more specialties may be represented. Here are the ones most commonly involved in normal, uncomplicated deliveries.

OBSTETRICIAN

An obstetrician, or OB, is a medical doctor who specializes in pregnancy and childbirth. A gynecologist, or GYN, specializes in women's reproductive health other than pregnancy and childbirth. An OB/GYN does both, and may even serve as a woman's primary care provider. Doctors are generally trained to be in charge, and you can expect an OB to take a more directive approach to managing your partner's pregnancy. An OB is authorized to handle complications that arise during labor and delivery, including performing C-sections. In an uncomplicated vaginal delivery, the OB is often not present during labor and arrives just in time to "catch" the baby as it's born.

CERTIFIED NURSE MIDWIFE (CNM)

A CNM is an advanced practice registered nurse who has post-graduate training in women's reproductive care and childbirth. You might think of a CNM as the nurse equivalent of an OB/GYN, but neither professional would be happy with that comparison. CNMs deliver babies in hospitals, birth centers and at home. Their scope of practice varies from state to state; in some places they practice with a medical doctor and in some places there are independent. They may or may not be able to do forceps or vacuum deliveries, and while they may assist at C-sections they don't make the incision. CNMs tend to take a more collaborative approach to managing pregnancy and birth. Their focus is uncomplicated pregnancy and delivery with minimal medical intervention.

OTHER KINDS OF MIDWIVES

Some midwives enter the field by paths other than nursing. They are not nurses and don't do hospital deliveries, focusing instead on birth center and home births. Certified midwives (CMs) complete post-graduate training on the same level as CNMs and take the same certification exam, although they are certified by a different professional board. Currently only a few states license CMs. Certified professional midwives (CPMs) meet their educational and practice criteria through apprenticeships or through midwifery schools, but don't have post-graduate degrees. Their scope of practice depends on state law and is less comprehensive than that of CMs. They are currently licensed in most but not all state. Lay midwives typically have no formal training, certification or licensing.

LABOR, DELIVERY AND POSTPARTUM NURSES

If your partner gives birth in a hospital, most of her care is likely to be provided by nurses who specialize in labor, delivery and postpartum care. These are the professionals who will be checking the fetal monitor and your partner's cervix, providing encouragement and nourishment and coordinating the rest of the care team. After the birth they will weigh and measure the baby, poke its heel for blood tests and give vaccines. They'll monitor your partner's recovery and offer assistance with bathing, diapering and breastfeeding.

LACTATION CONSULTANT

Babies and breasts are made to go together, but sometimes help is needed to get breastfeeding started. If your partner doesn't have friends or family members who have breastfed, she may just be unfamiliar with the process and need a little guidance. If she has inverted nipples, which point inward instead of outward, or if the baby has a cleft palate or other problem that interferes with feeding, a lactation consultant may be called in.

BIRTH ASSISTANT

If you choose a birth center or home birth with a midwife, you may also have a birth assistant. Sometimes the birth assistant is hired by the midwife, and sometimes you hire the birth assistant directly with the midwife's approval. A birth assistant is a professional who has the background and training to assist the midwife; they may be a nurse, or they may have specific birth assistant certification. If for some reason you are transferred to a hospital for the birth, an assistant you have hired directly might come along and serve as a doula.

DOULA

A doula serves more as a companion and as a knowledgeable, supportive friend than a healthcare provider. She (doulas are overwhelmingly female) will not be involved in the medical or nursing aspects, but will offer emotional and comfort care during pregnancy, labor and childbirth. The difference between a doula and you, the woman's partner, is that the doula will have done this before, and may have experienced it all herself, first hand.

ANESTHESIOLOGIST OR NURSE ANESTHETIST

If your partner opts for an epidural or other kind of numbing pain relief, this will be done by a medical doctor called an anesthesiologist or by an advanced practice nurse known as a nurse anesthetist. Once the epidural or other anesthesia is in place they will return to check it, but the moment-to-moment monitoring will be done by the labor and delivery nurses.

Chapter Thirteen
CHILDBIRTH METHODS AND GEAR

Giving birth is the most natural thing in the world, but it isn't easy. It's hard work, it hurts and things don't always go according to plan. Your partner may want all the medical interventions, or she may want to try to manage without them. Here's a quick roundup of the approaches you can choose from, and some of the equipment you can expect to have on hand during the birth.

LAMAZE

The Lamaze method, developed by a French obstetrician of the same name, was introduced in the US in the 1950s. Originally focused on breathing techniques, a typical Lamaze course now covers 12 hours of instruction and aims to teach the woman and her partner a number of strategies for being active, effective participants in the birth process. Lamaze acknowledges that a woman may opt for pain control, and that C-sections are sometimes necessary. As always, though, the goal is to minimize medical intervention.

. . .

Bradley

The Bradley method, also known as "husband-coached childbirth," was devised by an American obstetrician in the 1940s. Like Lamaze, it emphasizes that childbirth is a normal, natural process and encourages the woman and her partner to be active participants. The primary difference between Lamaze and Bradley is that while Lamaze offers ways to distract from the pain, Bradley teaches a relaxed acceptance of pain. The Bradley method also has a stronger emphasis on avoiding medical interventions.

Leboyer

In the 1970s Leboyer, another French obstetrician, introduced the radical notion that childbirth should take the baby's experience into account. He felt it was unnecessarily traumatic to pull a baby from its warm, cozy womb directly into a loud, cold, brightly-lit delivery room. As much as we may consider the baby's first cry as a triumphant confirmation of life, Leboyer saw it is a heartbreaking sign of the baby's distress. A Leboyer birth is quiet, dimly lit and, optimally, includes easing the baby into terrestrial life by delivering it into a warm bath, or placing it in a warm bath immediately after birth.

Water birth

Before its birth, a baby spends its entire life floating in warm, nourishing fluid. Many consider a water birth to be the most natural way possible to ease a newborn into life outside the womb. This can also be deeply soothing and relaxing for the woman, especially if she feels a special affinity for water. Being delivered into water is considered safe for the baby because it usually won't try to breathe until it leaves the water and is exposed to air. A water birth usually takes place in an inflatable tub, much like a child's backyard pool, made for the purpose. Water birth is contraindicated in some situations, such as if the woman has genital herpes or the baby is breech or there are other possible complications.

VAGINAL BIRTH AFTER CESAREAN (VBAC)

It was once considered too risky for a woman to attempt a vaginal delivery if she had a previous C-section. It was thought the woman's uterus might rupture where it had been cut before. Years of study have shown this is uncommon and that most women who have had a C-section can safely give birth vaginally afterward. This will depend, of course, on why the previous section was done. Some hospitals still consider VBAC unacceptably risky and won't allow it to be attempted under any circumstances.

GEAR FOR LABOR AND CHILDBIRTH

FETAL MONITOR

While the Doppler is great for doing a quick check on the baby's heart rate, more detailed information on how things are going is obtained with a fetal monitor, which also tracks the frequency and length of the woman's contractions. The most common kind of fetal monitor has two belts that wrap around the woman's belly, one for the baby's heartrate and one for contractions. If she has an epidural she'll stay in bed with the monitor on; otherwise, when she wants to get up and walk around, the monitor belts need to be taken off.

Less commonly, fetal monitoring may be done internally. With this method, a wired electrode is threaded through the woman's vagina and cervix and placed directly on the baby. Usually the baby's head is the part that is most readily available, and that's where the electrode goes; it's actually screwed into the baby's scalp. Optionally, a device called an intrauterine pressure catheter can be inserted into the uterus to measure the force of uterine contractions. This kind of monitoring allows the woman to move around more than if she had an external monitor, but less than if she had no monitor at all. Internal monitoring may be more accurate than external monitoring, but it does have some risks. Infection is one concern, and internal monitoring can't be used if the mother has herpes, HIV or hepatitis.

Birthing ball

A birthing ball, or birth ball, is just like the big exercise balls you use at the gym. Your partner can use one at home during pregnancy both as a comfortable place to sit and as a way to gently work the muscles in her back and abdomen. In labor, she may find it soothing to sit on the ball and bounce or rotate her pelvis in a circular motion. She can also put the ball either on the floor or on the bed and lean over it. It's possible to sit on the ball while in bed, but this can be tricky.

Peanut ball

A peanut ball is a little like two smaller birth balls joined in the middle. It's used like a birthing ball but is more stable and safer to use while in bed. This is especially true when the woman has an epidural; there's some evidence that using a peanut ball with an epidural helps keep labor progressing and makes a C-section less likely.

Birthing bar

A birthing bar, or squat bar, is a frame that can be

attached to the end of a bed. The woman can hold onto the bar or drape her arms over it while squatting.

Birthing stool

A birthing stool is a short stool that has the center cut out and an opening in the front, so that the seat is C-shaped. It takes the pressure off a woman's legs while she squats.

Forceps

There are different kinds of obstetrical forceps, but in general they look something like salad tongs. They are used when the baby's head is within reach but has stopped moving down, if it's turned in a way that's making it hard for it to negotiate the birth canal, or if changes in its heart rate indicate delivery needs to be sped up. Once the forceps are in place, the doctor or midwife can apply steady pressure while the woman pushes, helping to ease the baby out. If necessary, they can turn the baby's head. Forceps are pretty safe, although they may leave some minor bruises on baby's head and an episiotomy may be needed.

Vacuum extraction

Also known as vacuum-assisted delivery, with vacuum extraction a suction cup is applied to the top of the baby's head and a vacuum pump used to help pull the baby out. It's used for the same kind of reasons as forceps.

Chapter Fourteen

COMPLICATIONS IN LABOR AND CHILDBIRTH

PRETERM LABOR AND PREMATURE BIRTH

Labor that starts before the 37th week of pregnancy is called preterm labor, and a baby born this early is considered premature. In the past premature babies often didn't survive, but nowadays it isn't unusual for babies born at 25 weeks (and sometimes even earlier) to make it. The more premature a baby is, of course, the more medical care will be needed to help it mature enough to leave the hospital.

Sometimes Braxton Hicks contractions become increasingly intense in the last trimester and can be confused with preterm labor. Braxton Hicks contractions cause a generalized tightening of uterine muscles and some discomfort similar to mild menstrual cramps, but they don't cause the cervix to open. True labor contractions get increasingly painful, longer lasting and closer together. It's never wrong to check in with your partner's doctor or midwife if she isn't sure what kind of contractions she's having.

CERVICAL INCOMPETENCE

Also called cervical insufficiency or an incompetent cervix, this is when the cervix begins to thin and open too early in pregnancy, risking miscarriage or a premature delivery. Cervical incompetence isn't common. Some known or suspected risk factors include certain genetic disorders and having had a previous dilation and curettage (a procedure where the cervix is opened so the uterus can be accessed). Often there's no known risk factor.

Cervical incompetence typically doesn't cause any symptoms in the first trimester, but in the second trimester may feel a little like early labor, with pressure in the pelvis and vaginal spotting. If your partner is diagnosed with an incompetent cervix, various treatments may be tried to prevent premature labor or loss of the pregnancy. The most invasive treatment is called cervical cerclage, in which the cervix is actually sutured shut. The sutures are removed near the due date or when labor begins.

PREMATURE RUPTURE OF MEMBRANES (PROM)

A baby in the uterus floats in amniotic fluid, which is enclosed in the amniotic sac. The amount of amniotic fluid within the membranes increases until about 34 weeks, when there may be as much as 800 ml (about 27 ounces, or almost three-and-a-half cups). After that it starts to drop, until by 40 weeks there's about 600 ml of fluid.

The event popularly known as the woman's water breaking is the amniotic sac, or membranes, rupturing so the amniotic fluid escapes. This normally happens during labor, although in very rare cases babies are born with the membranes intact. PROM happens before labor starts, sometimes well before. The amniotic fluid may all empty at once, as it does on TV, or it may leak out slowly.

The pregnancy may be able to continue with a slow leak, as amniotic fluid is continually replaced, but the baby can't survive in the uterus without any fluid at all. When a great deal of fluid is lost through PROM, the baby will have to be delivered. If labor doesn't begin naturally, either it will be induced or the baby will be delivered by cesarean section.

SHOULDER DYSTOCIA

Dystocia means difficult childbirth, and shoulder dystocia is when birth is complicated by the baby's shoulders not fitting through the birth canal. Sometimes ultrasounds will offer advance warning of potential shoulder dystocia, and a cesarean section will probably be scheduled. Sometimes, though, the problem is unexpected and only becomes obvious after the baby's head is already out.

It might seem obvious that very big babies would be most likely to have shoulder dystocia, but most big babies don't have it, and most babies who do have it aren't exceptionally large. When shoulder dystocia does occur, the doctor or midwife will try a range of workarounds that may include changing the woman's position, performing an episiotomy, or manipulating the baby by reaching into the birth canal or pressing on it through the woman's abdomen. Fortunately these maneuvers are usually successful.

MECONIUM ASPIRATION

Even though a baby in the womb gets its nutrition through the placenta, by the second trimester it will begin swallowing amniotic fluid. Some of the fluid will be recycled as urine, which is part of why the volume of amniotic fluid increases.

Amniotic fluid contains more than just water, though; in addition to the discarded skin cells that make amniocentesis possible there may be lanugo, or fetal hair, and other bits and pieces. This organic matter accumulates in the baby's gut and forms its first poop, which is called meconium.

Normally meconium makes its appearance in the newborn's first few diapers, but sometimes it finds its way into the amniotic fluid before birth. This usually happens when the baby becomes distressed during labor, but sometimes there isn't any obvious reason for it.

If the baby swallows meconium, it can be pulled into the airway when it takes its first breaths. Often suctioning the airways is enough to keep problems from developing, but if the meconium makes its way down into the baby's lungs the baby may need to be admitted to the hospital for medical care.

STALLED LABOR

Labor is hard work, and at times your partner might wish it would stop. What she never wants before the baby comes, though, is for it to actually stop. Stalled labor is when contractions slow or stop altogether, or when they continue but without opening the cervix. This can be discouraging and exhausting, and increases the risk of ending up with a C-section.

Although the idea is outdated, many healthcare providers still believe that once a woman is in active labor, her cervix should open by at least 1 cm per hour. A midwife in a birth center or home birth may be willing to let a slow labor take its course (as long as mom and baby are okay), but in a hospital it will only be tolerated for so long before intervention is recommended.

It's important that you and your partner talk about your

commitment to vaginal delivery and make this clear in your birth plan. Recognize, of course, that things may not go as wished or planned, and that your feelings may change once things are underway. But decide ahead of time what kind of approach you want to take if labor stalls. Do you want to accept recommended medical interventions to keep things going? Or do you want to do whatever you can to avoid intervention?

What needs to be done to get stalled labor going again depends on what's causing it to slow.

WHAT YOU AND YOUR PARTNER CAN DO
Change position
Sometimes labor slows because the baby isn't in that ideal head-down, facing-mom's-spine position. She may be able to use a combination of gravity, walking and body movements to persuade the baby to settle into a better position. Even if she's in bed with an epidural, it's possible to help her move around. The midwife, doula, nurse or birth assistant will be able to suggest safe, effective movements and positions.

Nipple stimulation
Rubbing or kneading your partner's nipples may cause a release of oxytocin, a hormone that acts on the uterus. (In fact, if she was in danger of preterm labor she may have been told to avoid nipple stimulation for this reason.) This is something either you or she can do. Another good way for her to boost oxytocin release is to have an orgasm; this is something you might have tried at home if the baby was overdue and you wanted to get labor started. It's the rare woman who will be enthusiastic about this option while in labor—especially if she's in the hospital—but it might be worth consideration.

Check with midwife or nurse to make sure it's safe to try this option.

Take a shower

A warm shower can be very relaxing, and letting the water run over her breasts may provide some gentle nipple stimulation to get that oxytocin flowing.

What healthcare providers can do

If you are having a birth center or home birth, the midwife will help you with strategies to get a stalled labor going again naturally. If you are in a hospital, the go-to intervention is Pitocin, or augmented labor. Pitocin is a synthetic form of oxytocin that's infused intravenously. The advantage of Pitocin is that it's very effective at stimulating contractions. The disadvantage is that it can cause contractions that go from zero to excruciating in a very short time, sometimes leading to fetal distress or the need for labor-slowing pain relief. It's possible, though, for a carefully managed Pitocin infusion to mimic natural contractions.

Chapter Fifteen
THE BIRTH ITSELF

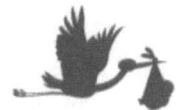

Back in the day, the laboring woman was whisked off to a private area and her partner was directed to the waiting room, where he paced and fretted, clutching a fistful of cigars, anxiously wondering if everything was okay. Eventually a doctor or nurse arrived at the door to inform him of the arrival of his son or daughter (surprise!) and invite him to visit his family.

Nowadays it's pretty much assumed you're going to be there to support your partner during labor, to witness the birth of your child and perhaps to have a hand in the proceedings. If you think pregnancy was a mental and emotional rollercoaster, wait until you experience childbirth!

LABOR

If everything you know about having babies comes from watching TV, you're in for a few surprises. A half-hour sitcom has to compress the entire process into just a few minutes, and it's much funnier when everything happens in a panicky rush. In reality, especially if this is your partner's first baby, you should expect least 24 hours to pass between the time your partner knows she's in labor to the sound of your baby's first cry. In fact, the earliest stage of labor, the part before you leave for the hospital or birth center or before the midwife arrives at your home, can take days.

It takes time

You may feel nervous and excited when labor begins, especially if you think it's going to be fast. After all the months of anticipation, it's go time! Then, as the hours go by, you may become worried, tired or even bored. If your partner has a doula or has asked another close friend of family member to be present, you may be able to take short breaks. Get something to eat, check your email, go for a walk (a short one!), catch your breath—then get back in there and support your partner.

Epidurals can be weird

If she has chosen to have an epidural, your partner may enter a kind of surreal situation where she sits comfortably in bed watching TV and playing cards, just as if it were any normal day. She'll have a fetal monitor strapped around her belly and the nurses will come in and look at the monitor to see how her contractions are going, because she won't be feeling them. You may be either relieved or bewildered by this turn of events. It can almost feel like you're literally waiting for a delivery—like someone else is getting the baby ready and you're just waiting for them to show up.

Otherwise, as your partner progresses through the stages of labor you can expect the action to get more intense and your attention (and hers!) to become much more focused. You might have been able to pop out for short breaks early on, but as she gets closer to pushing, and absolutely while she's pushing, you'll have to be fully present.

Push!

Once your partner's cervix is fully dilated and ready to let the baby through, she will finally be given the go-ahead to start pushing. This is likely to be a huge relief for her, as the urge to push can be overwhelming and she may have been fighting it up to that moment. She'll push during her contractions, which will by now be long and close together. This is very hard work! She may push for anywhere from a few minutes to a couple of hours. The baby's heart rate will be checked frequently and she can push as long as she needs to, provided she has the energy and the baby is okay. If she starts to tire, the baby isn't moving down or its heart rate indicates distress, possible interventions to speed up the delivery include episiotomy, forceps and vacuum extraction.

Crowning

At some point a doctor, midwife or nurse is likely to announce the baby is crowning, meaning the top of its head is clearly visible. This is an exciting development because the rest of the baby isn't far behind and birth is imminent. Depending on where you are, a mirror may be set up so your partner can see the baby's head crowning. This shows her that all is well and she's nearly done, which may be all the incentive she needs to power through the last few contractions.

If you are at the head of the bed with her, or supporting her from behind, you can watch in the mirror, too. If you are holding her hand but she doesn't want you any closer than that, you might find yourself looking directly at the emerging baby.

Either way, there's a lot to take in, and a lot of ways to feel about it. At this point your partner's vagina will not look anything like its usual self. It may be hard to believe it was once so inviting, or that it ever will be again. There will be stretching, and possibly tearing, and likely some bleeding. Pushing a small human being through the vagina also puts quite a strain on the neighboring rectum. If your partner didn't have visible hemorrhoids before, she might now. In fact, the inside of her rectum itself may put in an appearance. Many women poop a little while pushing. None of these things are unexpected and all become irrelevant once the baby comes.

Cesarean section

If your baby is delivered by cesarean, things will go a little differently. Your partner may have tried to deliver vaginally and ended up with an unexpected C-section, or it may have been planned in advance for various reasons. Either way, it will take place in a surgical suite. If your partner already has an epidural in place, it will provide the numbing she needs for the operation. Otherwise an epidural or other kind of numbing procedure will be used to make her comfortable. In very rare cases, if an epidural is not in place and the C-section is extremely urgent, general anesthesia may be used.

You will usually be allowed to stay with your partner for the C-section. It's still surgery, though, so you'll change into scrubs and may wear a surgical mask to wear over your nose and mouth or a cap to cover your hair. You'll be able to talk to and reassure your partner, and you'll await your baby's arrival together. As with a vaginal delivery, if the baby checks out okay it will be placed on mom's chest where you'll start getting acquainted while her incision is sutured.

THE NEWBORN

You may find your newborn baby to be the most miraculously beautiful thing you've ever seen, and fall head over heels in love at first sight. Or, you may find he or she looks like a gooey little extraterrestrial, and wonder how you will ever love him or her. Either reaction, or anything in between, is perfectly normal. Don't judge yourself if your feelings aren't immediately positive; sometimes the love grows slowly. But do keep any negative reactions to yourself. They might make for a funny story someday, but your partner doesn't want to hear it right now.

Some newborns are plump, clear-skinned and Instagram-ready. Some have red skin, angry faces and cone-shaped heads. They may be covered in a creamy biofilm called vernix, or lanugo, a kind of soft hair all over the body. If forceps or vacuum extraction were used, the head or face may be bruised. Again, all perfectly normal and not at all predictive of they will look like in the days to come.

A newborn is typically most alert in the first hour or two after birth. Your baby may yawn, squirm, grasp your finger, look at your face and recognize your voice. Your partner won't be making milk yet but will be encouraged to put the baby to her breast, which the baby should willingly do. Enjoy this time, because soon he or she will fall asleep and it may be a while before you get to interact like this again.

Assessing the newborn

The doctor or midwife attending the birth will be less concerned with your baby's good looks than with whether he or she looks good, health-wise. They will use the Apgar score to quickly determine if the baby has any problems that need addressing.

You may read that Apgar stands for "Appearance, Pulse, Grimace, Activity and Respiration," but that's just a memory aid. It's actually named after Virginia Apgar, the American doctor who invented it. An Apgar score is usually done at one minute and five minutes after delivery. The baby is given a score of 0, 1 or 2 on each of five criteria: heart rate, respiratory effort, muscle tone, reflexes and color. A score of 7 to 10 indicates a healthy baby who needs just routine care. A lower scores indicates continued monitoring is appropriate, and a very low or dropping score may mean it's time for medical intervention.

CUTTING THE CORD

The umbilical cord, the baby's lifeline up until birth, is no longer needed once the baby is breathing air. The cord contains two arteries that carried oxygen-rich blood and nutrients to the baby in the uterus, and one vein that carried depleted blood and waste away. Immediately after birth some transfer is still taking place, and you may notice the cord pulsing in time with your partner's heartbeat. As long as neither mom nor baby needs emergency care, there will be no rush to cut the cord; many midwives, especially, advocate for waiting for the pulsing to stop before cutting. Then they will put two clamps on the umbilical cord, cut in between the clamps, and place the baby on mom's chest. If you or your partner want to cut the cord, you'll be handed the scissors to do so. You may be surprised at how tough and gristle-like the cord is, so be ready. Not everyone wants to cut the cord; if you don't want to, just say no.

. . .

CORD BLOOD

Cord blood is the blood that remains in the placenta and the umbilical cord after the cord has been cut. It contains red and white blood cells, but it also contains the kind of blood-forming stem cells found in bone marrow. These stem cells, which can be used to treat a variety of life-threatening conditions, can be frozen and stored indefinitely. You can choose to donate your child's cord blood in the hopes it will be a good match for someone desperate for this kind of treatment, or you can pay to have it stored in case your family needs it in the future.

BREASTFEEDING

If your partner plans to breastfeed, she will be encouraged to start right away. She won't have milk yet—nor will the baby need it yet—but the oxytocin released when the baby latches on to her breast will stimulate her uterus to contract to its non-pregnant size. This is critically important to prevent excessive bleeding. The oxytocin and physical closeness also help promote bonding.

THE UTERUS

You may notice the doctor, midwife or nurse pressing on your partner's belly after the baby and placenta have both been delivered. They are feeling her uterus to make sure it's firm, so the blood vessels that were attached to the placenta are compressed. If the uterus doesn't clamp down on the blood vessels they can bleed heavily. If the uterus feels too soft, they may massage it by pressing on your partner's abdomen. If this isn't enough, the doctor or midwife may massage the uterus with one hand on the abdomen and one in the vagina. Pitocin, the synthetic oxytocin analog, may also be given. In the very unlikely case your partner's uterus doesn't respond to these measures, surgery may be needed.

EPISIOTOMY AND PERINEAL TEARS

You have probably wondered from time to time how it's even possible for a 7- or 8-pound baby to pass through your partner's vagina. No doubt your partner has spent some time thinking about this as well! What kind of magic makes it possible for her to pass a baby-size package through that small space?

Nature takes care of all of this, softening and loosening ligaments in the pelvis and lending elasticity to vaginal tissues so they can stretch and then return (or nearly return) to their pre-baby size. But skin and muscle can only stretch so far, and sometimes a baby needs a bit more space than mom's vagina can accommodate. Something has to give, and that something is her perineum.

The perineum is the space between the vagina and the anus. Sometimes the perineum will tear during childbirth, and sometimes the doctor or midwife will cut it. The cut is called an episiotomy. Healthcare practitioners may have strong opinions as to whether cutting or tearing is better. There are advantages and disadvantages to each.

Perineal tears may be minor or major. There are four degrees of tearing, depending on how many layers of tissue are involved and how far toward the rectum they go. One advantage of letting the perineum tear is that the least severe tear, which doesn't extend all the way to the muscle, is easier to repair and recover from than a cut that goes all the way through. The major disadvantage of letting the perineum tear is that the doctor or midwife has no control over how severe the tear turns out to be. A full thickness tear that reaches into the rectum can be a life-changing injury for the woman.

The main advantage of an episiotomy is that the doctor or midwife controls how far the cut goes. The main disadvantage is that the cut goes all the way through connective tissue and muscle and so may be more painful and take longer to heal than a superficial tear. There was a time when episiotomies were routine and nearly always done, but this is no longer the case.

If your partner has a perineal tear or episiotomy, some special care will be needed. A first degree tear doesn't usually need to be repaired, but an episiotomy or a more severe tear will need to be sutured. If she doesn't have an epidural in place she'll be given a local anesthetic to numb the area while the suturing is done. Afterward she'll be given a squirt bottle for cleaning and will need to monitor for signs of infection or other complications, just as she would for any other kind of incision or injury.

Even without tearing or cutting, your partner's perineum is likely to feel sore and a little fragile after a vaginal delivery. Childbirth is normal and natural, but that doesn't mean it's easy! When it's time to have a bowel movement she may feel like "everything is going to fall out" if she does any pushing. Applying counter-pressure to the perineum with a pad of toilet paper or gauze will help with this.

Chapter Sixteen
CESAREAN SECTION

As a rule, the female body is well-adapted to the task of delivering a baby through the birth canal, in what we call a vaginal delivery. The human species wouldn't have lasted as long as it has if procreation couldn't proceed naturally and without medical help.

That being said, vaginal delivery is sometimes not advisable and sometimes simply not possible. In these cases, the baby is delivered through cesarean section, commonly known as a C-section. In a C-section an incision is made through the woman's abdomen and into the uterus, and the baby is delivered through the incision. This is easier on mom and baby in some ways, but has its drawbacks as well.

Sometimes a C-section is planned and is scheduled for a particular date and time. The obvious advantage for you and your partner is that you know exactly when the baby is coming. Sometimes a vaginal delivery is planned but something occurs during labor that makes a C-section necessary. This may be worrisome or disappointing, but the aim is to ensure a healthy mom and baby.

REASONS FOR PLANNED C-SECTION

Breech or transverse baby

Late in pregnancy but before labor starts the baby usually "drops," or settles into position for birth. The ideal position is head down, facing mom's spine. A baby who settles with feet or butt down is called breech. Breech babies can be delivered vaginally, and many have been, but there are risks involved and nowadays many practitioners cannot or will not attempt them.

Some hospitals don't allow vaginal breech deliveries, and in some places breech births are considered high-risk and therefore outside the scope of a midwife's practice. A big concern is that in a breech birth the baby's head is delivered last, and unforeseen problems getting the head or shoulders through the birth canal could be disastrous.

A transverse baby is laying sideways, and obviously can't enter the birth canal like that. If efforts to persuade a transverse baby to turn are unsuccessful, a C-section will be necessary.

Genital herpes

Herpes may be an uncomfortable inconvenience for you and your partner, but for a newborn baby it can cause devastating neurological damage or even death. If your partner has contracted herpes late in pregnancy she won't have any antibodies to pass on to the baby, putting the baby at risk of an infection it can't fight off. If she contracted herpes well before this pregnancy her antibodies will help protect the baby. Nevertheless, if your partner has an active herpes outbreak as her due date approaches, a C-section will probably be recommended.

. . .

Mom's health problems

Some medical conditions can make vaginal delivery dangerous for a woman. These include heart and brain conditions that may be aggravated by the strain of pushing, and sometimes chronic or pregnancy-related conditions like diabetes or high blood pressure.

Obstructions

In placenta previa, the placenta has attached low in the uterus and completely or partially blocks the cervix. Fibroids, which are noncancerous growths that can develop in the uterus, can also obstruct the cervix. Sometimes there is an obvious mismatch between the size of the baby's head or shoulders and the mother's pelvic opening.

Previous C-section

If your partner has had a C-section before, she may be advised to have another one this time. It may be that the problem that led to the last C-section is still a problem. Also, there is a risk that during labor the uterus could rupture along the old incision, although this is less common with the way C-sections are done today.

A vaginal delivery after a C-section is called VBAC (vaginal birth after cesarean) and may or may not be advisable, depending on what kind of incision she had, how well she recovered and why it was done. About 60 percent to 80 percent of attempted VBACs are successful and result in a safe vaginal delivery, but some hospitals will not allow them anyway.

Multiple birth

Sometimes twins are delivered vaginally, if it looks like the delivery will be uncomplicated. If the position of one or both babies is problematic, a C-section may be scheduled for safety reasons. Triplets (or more!) are likely to be delivered by C-section because it's complicated to ensure the wellbeing of this many babies during labor and delivery.

REASONS FOR UNPLANNED C-SECTIONS

Fetal distress

If during pregnancy your partner notices the baby is not moving as much as usual, her doctor or midwife will check the baby's heart rate and possibly do an ultrasound. If these aren't reassuring a C-section may be advised. If the baby shows signs of distress during labor, such as a heart rate that is too fast, too slow or irregular, an emergency C-section may be done.

Pre-eclampsia

Pre-eclampsia, in which the woman develops high blood pressure and possible organ damage, that develops in the last trimester can sometimes reach crisis proportions as labor begins. The only definitive treatment for pre-eclampsia is to deliver the baby, so if it looks like it is progressing toward life-threatening eclampsia an emergency C-section will be done.

Labor is not progressing

An important reason not to rush to the hospital at the first sign of labor is that the clock starts ticking the minute your partner is admitted. At home or in a birth center a woman may be allowed to labor for days, but in a hospital there's an expectation that labor will progress along a fairly standard timeline. Otherwise, interventions to speed things along will be suggested, sometimes firmly.

If these are not successful, or if hours of intense contractions are simply not opening the cervix, at some point a C-section becomes inevitable. This is especially true if your partner's water has broken early on; this is known as premature rupture of membranes, or PROM, and presents a risk of infection if the baby isn't born in a timely manner.

Umbilical prolapse

This is when the umbilical cord, which the baby relies on for its oxygen, drops down into or through the cervix ahead of the baby. This can happen during labor but can also happen before labor begins, especially after PROM. Prolapse can cause compression of the umbilical cord, cutting off oxygen delivery to the baby. Depending on when it happens and how severe its effect on the baby, a C-section may be urgently needed.

Chapter Seventeen
COMPLICATIONS AFTER DELIVERY

UTERINE ATONY

*A*tony is a lack of muscle tone. The uterus is a muscular organ, and sometimes the way it is stretched and fatigued in pregnancy and childbirth can leave it lax and unresponsive. If this happens, the blood vessels where the placenta was attached to the lining of the uterus may continue to bleed. Your partner's uterus will be checked for firmness as soon as the placenta has been delivered. Normally it will be fine, and if it isn't a little massage is usually enough to get it started, but sometimes Pitocin is used. Some hospitals nowadays routinely give Pitocin to prevent atony.

HEMORRHAGE

Your partner will have bleeding after giving birth, regardless of whether she had a vaginal delivery or a C-section. This normal postpartum shedding of blood and tissue, called lochia, continues as the uterus contracts back down to its non-pregnant size and the cervix closes. It may be fairly heavy at first, with noticeable clots. The blood may pool up in her vagina when she's resting and come out all at once when she stands up. The bleeding should gradually get lighter until it stops altogether, which may take several weeks. Because the cervix is still partially open, putting anything in the vagina during this time risks introducing infection into the uterus, so tampons and intercourse are no-noes.

If for any reason your partner's uterus is slow to contract, she may have excessive bleeding, or hemorrhaging. Hemorrhage will be suspected if she has bright red blood for more than three days, if she passes very large clots or if she has symptoms of severe blood loss like feeling dizzy and clammy. It isn't very likely this will happen to your partner, but symptoms like these require medical follow up right away.

Chapter Eighteen
NOW YOU HAVE A BABY!

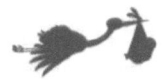

NEWBORN CARE IN THE HOSPITAL/BIRTH CENTER

If your baby is delivered in a hospital or birth center, the staff will have a few more tasks to perform while you and your partner celebrate and congratulate yourselves on a job well done.

HEEL STICK TEST

At some point a nurse will want to poke your baby's heel with a small lancet and squeeze out a few drops of blood onto a card. This card will then be sent off to a lab that will test for up to 30 different genetic conditions. The exact number of conditions tested for varies from state to state, but they all include certain conditions it's important to know about right away, like phenylketonuria (PKU). PKU is an inherited disorder that requires dietary treatment to prevent severe health problems. Another condition that is tested for, galactosemia, can potentially make breastfeeding dangerous for the baby, so it's important to know about it as soon as possible.

Weight and measurement

If your partner got regular prenatal care, and especially if she had any late ultrasounds, the measurements done after your baby is born will pretty much confirm what was already known. Your baby's length will be measured in inches; average length is 19 to 20 inches, although the normal range is more like 18 to 22 inches. Average weight is considered to be about 7.5 pounds, although anything from about 5.5 pounds to 10 pounds is considered normal. A newborn will usually lose a little water weight in the first few days, then start gaining again after that.

Hepatitis B vaccine

Newborns are routinely given a first hepatitis B vaccine, with two more to follow in the coming months. Hepatitis B is a virus that attacks the liver. An infant or young child who is infected with hepatitis B is at risk of becoming seriously ill and developing liver failure or cancer. If your partner has hepatitis B she can pass the virus on to the baby. In this case the baby will also need a dose of immune globulin to help fight off the infection.

As with other recommended vaccines you have the option of refusing this one. Just know that you don't have to be sexually active or a drug user to contract hepatitis B—the virus shows up in many people with no known risk factors, including children, and it can be transmitted by people who don't even know they have it. If you think you might refuse or postpone the hepatitis B vaccine, it's vitally important for your partner to be tested for it.

Vitamin K

Vitamin K, which is needed for blood clotting, doesn't cross the placenta very well and babies tend to be born without enough to protect them from excessive bleeding. They are at risk of vitamin K deficiency until they start eating solid food, usually around six months. An injection of vitamin K is recommended for every newborn to prevent bleeding during these first few months. Vitamin K can be given orally but it's less effective and requires repeated dosing. Breastmilk, while ideal for infant nutrition in nearly every way, doesn't contain much vitamin K. Infant formulas have vitamin K added but may not be sufficient if for any reason the baby doesn't get enough.

Erythromycin ointment

The practice of putting erythromycin ointment in the eyes of newborn babies became nearly universal once it was realized it could serious prevent eye infections in the first month of life. There are many agents of infection that can affect a baby's eyes, but the most serious are gonorrhea and chlamydia. All hospitals in the US will recommend the ointment, and in some states it's mandated by law. Some other countries have dropped the requirement in favor of screening pregnant women for sexually transmitted infections (STIs). There are many reasons to be checked for STIs in pregnancy, and this is another reason why prenatal care is so important.

Footprints, fingerprints and identity bands

Your baby may stay with you in your hospital room every minute from birth to discharge home, but you are likely to have at least short times apart. To be sure the right baby goes home with the right mom, the baby's footprints and mom's fingerprints are taken. Traditionally the prints have been done with ink on paper, but some places are introducing electronic scanners that take digital prints instead. Mom, baby and dad will be given matching ID bands to wear as well. Some hospitals place an electronic band on the baby's leg that will lock all the doors in the unit if the baby is taken too close to one of them. Any time a healthcare provider takes your baby out of your room, they should check ID bands when they come back. If they don't, speak up and remind them.

BATHING

Newborns can be a little messy right after they're born—they are dried off right away to keep them from getting chilled, but bits of blood and vernix, a creamy biofilm that forms on the skin in the womb, can stick to skin and hair. Hospital staff may offer to take your baby to the nursery for a bath or can help you do the bathing in your room. You may also choose *not* to bathe your baby yet. Any vernix that remains can be rubbed in instead of washed off, as it forms a protective barrier on the skin.

MORE NEWBORN CARE

UMBILICAL STUMP

After the umbilical cord is cut a portion of it, called the stump, remains attached to the baby. At first there will still be a plastic clamp on the stump, which will make it especially awkward. The clamp is to prevent bleeding through the stump until its blood vessels shut down completely. Once the cord is dry the clamp can be removed, generally within the first day or so. The stump, however, will remain for another two or three weeks, slowly shrinking and shriveling until it finally falls off, leaving behind your baby's cute little belly button. You'll have to keep the stump clean, diaper around it and watch for signs of infection. Fortunately, infection is uncommon; unfortunately, oozing of stinky goo is not. You and your partner will be given instructions on how to tell the difference between normal decay of this formerly living tissue and infection that needs treatment.

Jaundice

Jaundice is a yellowing of the skin, and sometimes of the eyes, that is caused by a buildup of bilirubin. Bilirubin is a component of red blood cells that is released when old cells are broken down to make way for new ones, a process that goes on continuously in all of us. In the uterus, the baby's bilirubin is cleared through the placenta. After birth, the baby's liver needs to take over this function, but there can be a delay before it reaches full capacity. During this time even healthy full-term babies can become mildly jaundiced. Usually keeping the baby well-fed and spending some time in sunlight, even next to a window, is sufficient. More significant jaundice may require treatment with special lights, and in some cases with IV fluids. In rare cases severe jaundice signals serious medical conditions that require aggressive medical management. You'll be given lots of information on how to monitor your baby for jaundice.

Circumcision and the Foreskin

Certainly you and your partner will have discussed whether or not you want your son to be circumcised, and hopefully you were in agreement! There was a time when male circumcision, whether just after birth or later, routine or ceremonial, was nearly universal in the US, but now many parents are choosing to forgo it. There are health, hygiene and cosmetic considerations as well as religious and family traditions to weigh, but in the end the choice is up to you. If you decide against circumcision, you'll need to learn about caring for your son's penis and foreskin. At birth the foreskin will be attached to the glans, or head of the penis. In time it will separate and can be retracted, but this could take anywhere from hours to years. Until then it should never be forcefully retracted, and you should only "clean what is seen." If you decide to go ahead with circumcision it can be done before you leave the hospital or, if your son was born outside a hospital, in the pediatrician's office. This is a relatively minor procedure but will require some aftercare to keep your son comfortable and prevent infection. If you have your son circumcised by a mohel, oral suction to remove the foreskin is strongly discouraged as it can transmit infection.

GOING HOME

The day has finally come! This is an exciting time for your new family! If you had your baby in a hospital, how long you stay before going home depends on whether your partner had a vaginal delivery or a C-section, and how well she and the baby are doing. If all is well and there are no complications, you can expect to head home in a day or two after a vaginal delivery and three or four days after a C-section.

Car seat

You'll be expected to provide a safe, properly fitting infant car seat for the for the ride home, so don't forget it! Make sure you've practiced putting it in and taking it out of the car so you don't have to figure it out in real time.

Visitors

The arrival of a new baby is an exciting time, and your friends and family will want to drop by to check out the newcomer and wish you well. There will be plenty of time for this, though, and it doesn't have to happen all at once. If you've been on an adrenaline high since the baby was born, you can be sure the crash is coming. All three of you need rest and nourishment. There is usually a bit of a honeymoon period when a newborn baby sleeps a lot and cries very little, and you will begin to think you have been blessed with the happiest, most chill kid ever. That isn't going to last, though, so sleep while you can.

You'll want to limit the number of visitors you have each day, how long they stay and the number that are present at one time. If they don't offer to bring food, wash dishes or run a load of laundry, ask them to do so. Anyone you can't be this direct with can wait to visit until you and your new family are more settled and can accommodate them.

Be ready to gently refuse entry to anyone who has a cold or any other contagious illness, no matter how minor. Yes, your baby will need exposure to germs to build a healthy immune system, but that's for later, when his or her immune system has kicked in. Ask any visitor, even family, who wants to hold your baby to wash their hands first. Don't forget to stock up on hand sanitizer! And kissing is definitely out; as much as visitors may want to smooch those chubby little cheeks, exposure to the herpes virus at this age can be disastrous.

Chapter Nineteen
BABY CARE AT HOME

At last, you're home. Visitors have departed, the house is quiet, and it's just you, your partner, and your new baby. Suddenly, it hits you: you've never done this before. What happens next? You've read all the books, watched all the videos and listened while friends and family gave you their best advice. But now that it's all real, you may feel a little overwhelmed.

Don't worry.

Whether you're on top of the world or scared to death, what you're feeling is perfectly normal. Sure, this is the most important project you'll ever take on. But you've got lots of time to figure things out and grow into the role. You'll get some things wrong, but you'll get many things right. Just be patient with yourself and your new little family. You got this.

CARING FOR YOUR NEWBORN

Basically, newborn babies eat, sleep and poop. Oh, and cry. That's pretty much it. Let's look at each of those.

. . .

EATING

Breastfeeding

Whatever other purposes they serve before and after, with a baby in the house breasts are for milk. Not every woman will breastfeed, of course; your partner may have reasons not to, and fortunately there are alternatives. But if she does, this will bring its own set of advantages and challenges.

The advantages are many. Breastfeeding:

- Meets baby's nutritional needs perfectly
- Leads to very mild-smelling baby poop
- Releases oxytocin, encouraging mother-baby bonding
- Stimulates mom's uterus to contract and return to non-pregnant size
- Lowers mom's risk of breast and uterine cancers
- Is super convenient!

There may be challenges, as well. Breastfeeding:

- Is natural but doesn't always feel natural at first
- Can be uncomfortable when nipples are tender or when breasts are engorged
- Requires mom to pump if she needs to be away from the baby
- Can feel awkward or even be discouraged in public places
- Limits what mom can wear, as breasts need to always be accessible
- Can make dad feel left out

BOTTLE FEEDING

Bottles make it possible for the baby to be fed if your partner needs to return to work or otherwise needs to be away, or if she isn't breastfeeding. A lot of research has gone into designing bottle nipples that babies find acceptable, and you may need to try a couple of different ones. Whether breastmilk or formula is in the bottle, being able to hold and feed your baby can help you enjoy the kind of bonding you might otherwise miss out on.

SLEEPING

Immediately after birth your baby will probably have an hour or two of quiet alertness, then fall asleep. Every newborn is unique, of course, but many will then go on to stay relaxed and sleep pretty much full-time for the next couple of weeks. Then, for the next few months, a baby sleeps about 17 out of every 24 hours. They usually wake up hungry every three or four hours, but breastfed babies often nurse for comfort, too, and may wake up wanting the breast even more often.

You may be tempted to tiptoe around, whispering and keeping the house perfectly quiet while your baby is sleeping, but this isn't necessary. First of all, there's a reason we use the expression "sleep like a baby." They're pretty good at it. Babies need to sleep, and yours will adapt to the ambient sound level. Better to live your normal life—within reason, of course. Excessive noise isn't good for anyone.

A good rule when you have a little one—for your partner, certainly, but also for you—is to sleep when the baby sleeps. It's tempting to try to get as much done as possible when the baby is otherwise occupied, and this is fine for you if it helps you feel less stressed. But put off whatever you can. The responsibilities of daily life will always be there, but your hours of uninterrupted sleep are limited. This is especially true for your partner, who needs to be encouraged to rest as much as possible.

POOPING

Your newborn came preloaded with poop called meconium. Meconium is made up of amniotic fluid, discarded skin cells and other bits of waste your baby ingested in the womb. You can expect to see meconium, which is thick and tarry, in your baby's diapers for the first few days before the transition to normal poop.

One of the advantages of breastfeeding is that the baby's poop, until solid foods are introduced, is pale in color and has a mild, inoffensive odor. Be prepared, though—there is likely to be lots of it. A baby who gets formula will have poop that is darker in color, thicker and has a stronger smell. Either way, between peeing and pooping you can expect to go through at least 10 diapers a day.

Disposable diapers are easy to deal with, but most are made with plastic that will be landfill for generations to come. Biodegradable diapers are available, although they may be expensive. Cloth diapers are pretty messy to deal with and it can be argued that the laundering they require isn't environmentally kind, either. One nice thing about cloth diapers is you can hire a service to bring you clean ones and take the soiled ones away. Some parents use cloth diapers at home and disposables away from home.

Similarly, you can buy wet wipes for diaper-change cleaning or use washcloths, or use some combination of the two.

CRYING

Just about when you and your partner start high-fiving over how well you're handling this whole parenting thing and how lucky you are to have this easy baby, everything changes big time! Your sweet, happy baby has been possessed by a demon spirit that can't be soothed or placated. Crying jags go on for hours, no matter how often you feed, change diapers, burp or walk the halls. You're frustrated, sleep-deprived and sometimes you feel irrationally angry. What's happening?

At around two weeks, normal newborns enter what's been termed the Period of **PURPLE** Crying. The letters stand for:

Peak of crying. The crying starts around two weeks, peaks in the second month, then tapers off over months three to five.

Unexpected. There's no rhyme or reason to when the crying starts.

Resists soothing. Nothing you do makes any difference.

Pain-like face. The baby looks to be in pain, but isn't.

Long-lasting. The baby may cry for five hours a day . . . or more.

Evening. Crying is most likely in the late afternoon or evening, even if the baby was perfectly happy all day.

As awful as this period is, it is normal and it does end as the baby's nervous system matures.

This is the time in a baby's life when they are most at risk of being injured by an angry, exhausted parent. You may be horrified to feel rage bubbling up inside you as endless crying pushes you closer to the edge. If you are in danger of losing control, or if you just need a break, this is the time to hand the baby off to your partner or other calmer adult and go for a walk. By taking care of yourself first, you will be the in best form to take care of your child. In fact, there's nothing wrong with gently laying the baby down in a crib, bassinet or other safe place, closing the door and walking away. Not for a long time—you aren't going to neglect your baby or give up on trying to soothe them. But it's better to walk away for a few minutes and catch your breath than to risk harming them.

BATHING

Your newborn doesn't need much cleaning beyond the diaper area. The umbilical stump should be kept as dry as possible to prevent infection, so if more than bottom-wiping is needed it's best to stick with sponge bathing until it falls off. After that you can do full baths in a baby tub or any container that's big enough for a baby and some water. Lots of parents use the kitchen sink; just be sure to clean it well, both before and after.

Unless the baby is sweaty or poopy you can just wash with plain water. If you need a little more cleaning power you can use any gentle, mild-smelling soap; it doesn't have to be a special baby product. And you can use one soap on both head and body at this age; shampoo can wait until you've got a full head of hair to work with. Your baby is likely to be very relaxed in a warm bath, which probably brings back happy memories of floating snug and carefree in the womb. Just remember they can't breathe underwater anymore and need to be protected from getting chilled.

UMBILICAL STUMP

The umbilical cord was living tissue, and the stump left behind after the cord is cut is living tissue that dies. It will shrivel up and turn black, and a small amount of fluid may leak from the point where it joins your baby's still-living skin. You'll be given instructions on how to care for it. Basically, you'll wipe away any poop that gets on it and try to keep diapers from rubbing against it (disposable diapers for newborns often leave a space in front for this reason).

Parents used to be told to apply rubbing alcohol to the stump, but this isn't really necessary. Infection is rare but you'll want to check in with your baby's healthcare provider if you notice redness, swelling or a smelly discharge.

VAGINAL DISCHARGE

Sometimes a newborn baby girl will have a little vaginal discharge, either light in color or even a little bloody. Her vulva may also appear red and swollen. This is caused by exposure to mom's hormones before she was born and will gradually clear up.

FORESKIN CARE

If your baby boy has an intact foreskin, it probably won't be very moveable at first. Just wash around it ("clean what's seen") and never use force to retract it. If he's already been circumcised, you'll have been given care instructions.

IF YOU'RE interested in learning more about newborn care, check my books "Easy Newborn Care Tips" - Proven Parenting Tips For Your Newborn's Development, Sleep Solution And Complete Feeding Guide, *and* "Newborn Care Basics"- Baby Care Tips For New Moms.

You will find plenty of tips and effective solutions for caring to your baby.

Chapter Twenty
PARENTAL CARE AT HOME

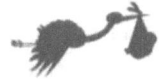

On the one hand, pregnancy and childbirth are normal, natural parts of life and women do it every day. On the other hand, creating new life and bringing it forth into the world is like having the greatest superpowers ever, and doing it makes your partner a superhero.

Just as some women seem to breeze through pregnancy while others endure nine of the most miserable months of their life, some will be up and fully active right after giving birth while others will undergo an extended period of slow recovery. Your partner will probably fall somewhere in the middle. She's been through a lot, and she deserves some consideration, even more so if there were complications along the way.

With all this attention on your partner's needs, you may feel at times like your own needs are being overlooked, and that's likely to be true for a while. But as your partner recovers from the physical stress of childbirth and you both get better at handling the demands of parenthood, this will get better. You will have a social life again, you'll be able to focus on your career and you'll even get to enjoy time to yourself. Maybe not as much as before—but the trade-off will be well worth it.

HER EMOTIONS

It's impossible to predict what your partner's emotional state will be just after the baby is born. Certainly the amount of support she has, and the amount of sleep she's getting, will have a big influence, as will the continuing ebb and flow of hormones. Overall, a mix of positive and negative emotions is to be expected, as with any major life change. It's very common, though, for new mothers to have a range of bad feelings they may find hard to talk about. Some celebrities are helping overcome the stigma of postpartum mood disorders by openly sharing their own experiences.

POSTPARTUM BLUES

It's estimated that up to 90 percent of all women experience some degree of "baby blues." The blues generally kick in a couple of days after birth, peak within the next few days and then gradually resolve over about two weeks. Your partner may have times when she feels sad, frustrated or angry. She may cry easily and have doubts about her mothering abilities. These feelings come and go, resolve with sleep, exercise or emotional support, and alternate with times when she feels happy and optimistic.

POSTPARTUM STRESS SYNDROME

The next step up in severity is postpartum stress, which may afflict up to 75 percent of all new mothers. If your partner has postpartum stress she may appear to be coping well, while inside she is eaten up with anxiety and sadness.

She may feel disappointed in herself, her baby and the experience of motherhood, and she may worry she isn't up to the job. She may find it very hard to admit she's having these feelings, as that would feel like proof she's not good enough. Hopefully you know your partner well enough to recognize the signs of stress and can offer extra support to help her get through it. Encourage her to talk about her feelings, either to you or to a trusted friend or family member.

Postpartum depression

Postpartum depression affects up to one in every four new mothers. Postpartum depression can be sneaky, either coming on early like postpartum blues or not rearing its ugly head until 18 months later. This form of depression runs much deeper than the blues and can completely destroy your partner's self-esteem and ability to take any pleasure in her baby or her life. If your partner suffers postpartum depression, she may have thoughts of harming herself or the baby—she needs professional care, urgently. She should start with her own healthcare provider to rule out medical conditions that could be contributing to her depression.

Postpartum anxiety

Closely related to postpartum depression and sometimes going along with it is postpartum anxiety, which affects up to one in 10 women. This is not the normal anxiety that comes with being a first-time parent. Sometimes the anxiety is generalized, and sometimes it manifests as postpartum panic disorder or postpartum obsessive compulsive disorder. Women who have experienced anxiety before having a baby are most at risk. Professional help may be needed.

. . .

Postpartum psychosis

Fortunately, postpartum psychosis is rare; this severe mental illness is estimated to affect only one or two out of every 1,000 new mothers. Women who were diagnosed as bipolar before pregnancy are at the greatest risk, but any woman can be affected. Psychosis is a break with reality. In the unlikely event your partner experiences postpartum psychosis she may have frightening mania, crippling depression or both. She may also suffer terrifying delusions and hallucinations, putting her, the new baby and any other children she has in grave danger. Postpartum psychosis is an emergency and requires immediate medical care.

YOUR EMOTIONS: PATERNAL POSTNATAL DEPRESSION

Yes, it can happen to you, too. You might not be experiencing the same hormone flow and body changes as your partner, but you are also worrying, stressing and losing sleep. You may be dismayed to find the happiness wearing off and the reality of becoming a father weighing heavily on you. This is incredibly normal; estimates are that up to one in every four new fathers experience some degree of postpartum mood disorder.

If it happens to you, make sure you're getting some time *you* time. Go out for a run or bike ride, or meet up with the guys for a little basketball or a celebratory beer. If you find nothing makes you feel better, don't be afraid to get professional help.

HER VAGINA

It's been through a lot. If you watched your baby being born you may have doubted your partner's vagina could ever be its old self again, but it's amazingly resilient and will bounce back in time.

After a vaginal delivery she will have bleeding for up to six weeks and her cervix will need time to close completely. Intercourse during this time is not recommended due to the risk of uterine infection. If she had perineal tearing or an episiotomy she will feel pretty sore. Typical comfort measures include ice packs followed by sitz baths, which basically means soaking in a warm bath. She may be advised to encourage healing by laying on the bed with her legs apart and aiming a lamp at the area.

HER BELLY

Some women are surprised to find they still look pregnant after the baby has been born. This may be partly due to weight put on during pregnancy, and partly to the stretching and softening of the abdominal muscles. Your partner may notice very distinct separation of the rectus abdominis, the "six pack" muscles. This is called diastasis recti and usually resolves with time, although in some women the abdominis never fully fuse again.

If your partner had a C-section she will probably have a horizontal incision low on her abdomen. This is known as a "bikini cut" because it's low enough to stay hidden under bikini bottoms. The old school vertical cut up the center of her abdomen is rarely done anymore. Her incision may have been sutured or stapled; staples make for a quick and convenient repair but sutures are less likely to lead to infection or other complications.

If your partner has stretch marks they may be red or purple now. They will fade in color over time and may nearly disappear.

HER BREASTS

Although they likely grew larger and heavier during pregnancy, your partner's breasts won't actually start producing milk right after the baby is born. She will produce a creamy, nutrient-rich pre-milk called colostrum, though, and the colostrum along with the baby's body fat and fluids accumulated in the womb will carry it through until her milk comes in.

Within a few days her breasts may fill with milk suddenly, becoming large, hard and very tender; this is called engorgement. The best treatment for engorgement is a hungry baby! At first her breasts may fill with far more milk than the baby can drink, and she may be tempted to relieve the pressure by pumping or expressing (pressing with the hands) the excess milk. This can be done just a little if she's really miserable or if her breasts are so hard the baby is having trouble latching on, but it's best to resist the temptation as it gives her breasts the message that more milk is needed. Within a few days her milk supply will adapt to the baby's appetite and everyone will be happier. If your partner isn't going to be breastfeeding, her milk will still come in and she'll be given instructions on how to proceed.

CONCLUSION

Becoming a parent for the first time is an experience that brings happiness and fear simultaneously. Pregnancy is a glorious time leading to a miracle of producing a new life from a cell. However, the adventure of pregnancy and parenthood has its high and lows, but an experience every individual would relish. Men play a vital role in both conception and the upcoming experience. The role of a father is significant even during pregnancy. Both moms and dads have nine months to prepare themselves for looking after the baby and getting everything ready to welcome the new member. Before that, they also have to prepare themselves for the journey of pregnancy.

The pregnancy phase is more foreign to men in contrast to managing a newborn baby. Men must understand that women go through a lot of challenges like nausea, vomiting, morning sickness, heartburns and indigestion, tiredness, and back pain. Apart from it, they experience mood swings due to hormonal changes in the body. Hence, expectant dads need to be as supportive as possible from an emotional as well as physical perspective. Besides, you will not feel excluded at any time if you will contribute to activities like shopping, visiting doctors, birth planning, and so on. Even though doing all these can be overwhelming, this guide has done well in simplifying these experiences to help you enjoy fatherhood.

The initial step after hearing the good news is to visit a professional and take advice about the precautionary measures. The chances of miscarriage are higher in the early phase of pregnancy and the awkward bits are also greater in the first trimester. The mother must eat well for the nourishment of the baby and exercise regularly to prepare the body for pregnancy and childbirth. You can support your partner by doing physical exercises with her. Furthermore, she can have a craving for food at any time of the day, so you need to be prepared for that.

Preparation of the home to welcome the baby and the financial planning are also important phases when expecting a child. Carefully go through the section that highlights this area and make sure every step is put to use.

This book offers insights not only on the medical aspects of pregnancy but also on the social, and economic factors. You are prepared to make a feasible financial plan and savings account for your child. Moreover, you also got the idea of what changes can be made to the house to provide a safe environment for the baby.

You have gained detailed information about prenatal care, the issues, and complications related to each phase of pregnancy as well as childbirth. Having information makes it easier for you to ensure that your partner receives appropriate prenatal care. A healthy lifestyle and good prenatal care are the best protection mechanisms against pregnancy complications. Nonetheless, labor and childbirth are crucial phases; hence, concise and adequate information has been provided to educate you about the peculiarities of labor and

CONCLUSION

childbirth. In this way, you will be ready to be there for your wife and know what to expect. After delivery complications were discussed to inform you about the unfortunate possibilities, you have gained experience that will enable you take necessary actions that will help your partner.

Now, the baby has arrived, meaning that your responsibility increased. You have become aware of the important tests that are done right after birth and vaccines given to the baby. When finally coming home, having a large number of guests or guests with cold or contagious diseases is definitely prohibited. The baby has a weak immune system, which means you need to be careful about who is kissing or touching your baby.

Your partner will be exhausted from all the labor and delivery process, as well as handling the baby is a new thing for her also, just like you. As highlighted, the mother will be also going through a major life change; she might be experiencing a combination of positive and negative emotions. At this time, your support is very important and it can be provided by taking turns to take care of the baby at night, bathing the baby, or changing the diapers and clothes. Not only do mothers experience postpartum depression, you can also suffer from paternal postnatal depression. You might be stressing and worrying about the reality of fatherhood. If something like this happens, make sure that you give your self some "me" time. Go out somewhere to be relaxed and stress-free. However, if the problem persists, get some professional help.

Whether you believe you are ready or not, you have started the journey. You have to cherish the journey because not all people have the opportunity to experience this wonderful event in their lives. You can prepare yourself by absorbing the information you have gained from the book and make this experience as much delightful as possible. Just be present in your partner and baby's lives and you will surely have a great experience of pregnancy and parenthood.

Don't worry! It is impossible that all things are going to be perfect because you will make mistakes like everyone. You will also have moments of parenting brilliance. The book aims to rectify the probability of mistakes to make the journey enjoyable. Nonetheless, you and your partner will find the rewards for the sacrifices and hard work you both are putting in.

It seemed like you have to learn and think a lot about many things – and honestly, you have to! But you will figure it out like all the dads before you. You have time to get ready before the baby arrives, and a lot of years ahead to get used to the parenting strategies. Get ready to have an adventurous journey and enjoy every moment of it.

Forget about being perfect, just be there for your partner and baby in the best way possible. You will find your way and the experience easier as you prepare yourself by reading this helpful guide on becoming a dad.

Congratulations!

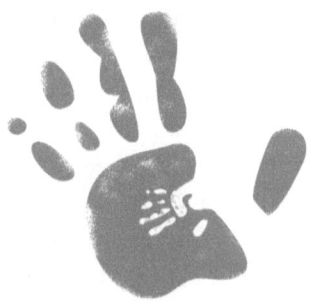

THANK YOU

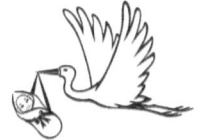

Before you leave, I just want to tell you how I have appreciated your effort of buying and reading the whole book.

If you also liked this book, please, **tell me what you liked the most leaving a review on the store where you purchased it**...It'd mean the world to me! Also, your review would help other customers make an informed purchase.

I hope you've gained fruitful tips and information that can be implemented in your experience and facilitate you to be an awesome partner and dad during pregnancy and childbirth. The management of a newborn is the easy part of parenting, the hard part is to imparting the right values, teaching them good habits, and making them a good human being.

Thanks again,
Lisa Marshall
& Johnny Antonelli

ALSO BY LISA MARSHALL

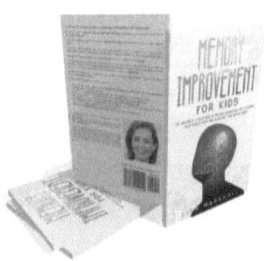

Memory Improvement For Kids

The Greatest Collection Of Proven Techniques For Expanding Your Child's Mind And Boosting Their Brain Power

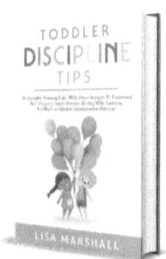

Toddler Discipline Tips

The Complete Parenting Guide With Proven Strategies to Understand And Managing Toddlers' Behavior, Dealing With Tantrums, And Reach An Effective Communication With Kids

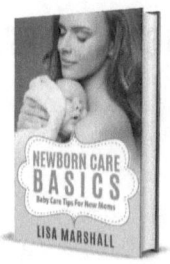

Newborn Care Basics

Baby Care Tips For New Moms

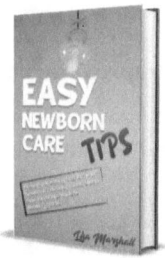

Easy Newborn Care Tips

Proven Parenting Tips For Your Newborn's Development, Sleep Solutions And Complete Feeding Guide

www.ingramcontent.com/pod-product-compliance
Lightning Source LLC
Chambersburg PA
CBHW020417080526
44584CB00014B/1368